The Sun's Touch: The Impact of Solar Flares on Human Health

Aeron P. White

Aeron P. White

ISBN-13: 979-8-3282-5186-0

Aeron P. White

For my mother, Norah, because she loves the Sun so much.

For my daughter, Rebecca, hoping that this book gives her necessary insight for a healthy future under the Sun.

For my grandson, Albi-Brian, and future unborn grandchildren, hoping their future is a little more secure with insight from this book.

CONTENTS

ACKNOWLEDGMENTS

Thanks go to ChatGPT4o for valuable research material.

Thanks to all of the researchers who have contributed to this area of research.

Thanks to my wife, Rita, for listening objectively and critically but also for believing in my intuitive insight when we discussed the topic of this book many times over the past 10 years.

1 FOREWORD

The sun, our closest star, has always fascinated humanity. From ancient civilizations that worshipped it as a deity to modern scientists who study its intricate behaviors, the sun remains a central figure in our understanding of the universe and our place within it. Its light and warmth are essential for life on Earth, but its dynamic and sometimes volatile nature also poses challenges and risks that we are only beginning to fully comprehend.

This book, "The Sun's Touch: The Impact of Solar Flares on Human Health" is a timely and comprehensive exploration of how solar phenomena, particularly geomagnetic storms and their associated solar flares and Coronal Mass Ejections (CMEs), affect human health and societal infrastructure. The detailed examination presented in these pages underscores the necessity of understanding and preparing for the diverse impacts of solar activity.

Our journey into this subject begins with the fundamental mechanisms of solar activity. The sun, far from being a static ball of gas, is a dynamic entity with a highly active magnetic field. Solar flares and CMEs are manifestations of this magnetic energy being released into space. When these events occur, they can propel vast quantities of charged particles and radiation toward Earth. The interaction of these solar emissions with Earth's magnetic field can lead to geomagnetic storms, which have the potential to disrupt modern technological systems and, as emerging research suggests, impact human health.

The historical context provided by significant events such as the Carrington Event of 1859 and the Quebec blackout of 1989 illustrates the profound effects that geomagnetic storms can have. These events not only caused technological disruptions but also raised questions about their impact on human health, leading to the burgeoning field of research we explore in this book.

The detailed chapters on the cardiovascular and

neurological effects of geomagnetic storms delve into the ways in which these solar events can influence human physiology. The correlations between increased geomagnetic activity and higher incidences of heart attacks, strokes, mood disorders, and sleep disturbances are compelling. The potential mechanisms, including disruptions in heart rate variability, blood pressure, brain wave patterns, and hormone levels, provide a foundation for understanding how external electromagnetic fields might interact with biological systems.

One of the most intriguing areas of research is the influence of geomagnetic storms on hormone regulation, particularly melatonin and serotonin. These hormones are critical for regulating sleep and mood, respectively. Disruptions in their production and balance can lead to significant health consequences, highlighting the importance of further research in this area.

Radiation exposure, especially for astronauts and high-altitude pilots, is another critical concern. The increased radiation levels during geomagnetic storms pose risks such as DNA damage, cancer, and acute radiation syndrome. The development of advanced shielding materials and pharmaceutical countermeasures is essential for protecting those most vulnerable to these effects.

The societal and economic impacts of geomagnetic storms are equally significant. Power grid failures, communication disruptions, and navigation system malfunctions can have widespread and costly repercussions. Protecting critical infrastructure through technological advancements and regulatory standards is paramount for maintaining societal stability.

Public health preparedness and public awareness are also vital components of resilience. Educating healthcare providers and the general public about the potential health impacts of geomagnetic storms can lead to better preparedness and response strategies. Community engagement and public education campaigns can enhance societal resilience by promoting informed and proactive behaviors.

Looking ahead, this book underscores the need for continued interdisciplinary research. Understanding the precise mechanisms through which solar activity impacts human health requires collaboration between space scientists, medical researchers, engineers, and social scientists. Longitudinal studies and innovative research methods will provide deeper insights into the chronic effects of geomagnetic storms and inform the development of effective protective measures.

Technological innovation will also play a crucial role in enhancing resilience. Advanced monitoring and early warning systems, improved radiation shielding, and wearable health technologies are just a few examples of how we can protect ourselves from the effects of solar activity. Additionally, policy development and international collaboration are essential for addressing the global nature of geomagnetic storms and ensuring a coordinated response.

In conclusion, " The Sun's Touch: The Impact of Solar Flares on Human Health" offers a comprehensive and insightful exploration of the complex interactions between solar activity and our biological and technological systems. By integrating knowledge from various scientific disciplines and advancing our understanding of these phenomena, we can better prepare for and mitigate the impacts of solar activity. This book serves as a valuable resource for researchers, healthcare professionals, policymakers, and anyone interested in the dynamic relationship between our sun and life on Earth. As we continue to explore and understand the powerful forces of our nearest star, we move closer to ensuring a safer and more resilient future for all.

2 INTRODUCTION

The sun, our nearest star, is a dynamic and powerful celestial body that profoundly impacts life on Earth. Beyond providing the light and warmth necessary for life, the sun also influences our planet through its magnetic activity. This activity includes solar flares and Coronal Mass Ejections (CMEs), which are significant bursts of solar wind and magnetic fields rising above the solar corona or being released into space. When these solar events interact with the Earth's magnetosphere, they can trigger geomagnetic storms that affect not only our technological systems but also potentially our health.

Understanding the effects of CMEs and solar flares on human physiology and biochemistry is a fascinating and complex subject. These solar phenomena release vast amounts of energy and charged particles into space. When directed towards Earth, they can disturb the Earth's magnetosphere, leading to geomagnetic storms. While the immediate technological impacts, such as satellite disruptions, power grid failures, and communication disturbances, are well-documented, the potential impacts on human health are less understood and constitute a burgeoning field of research.

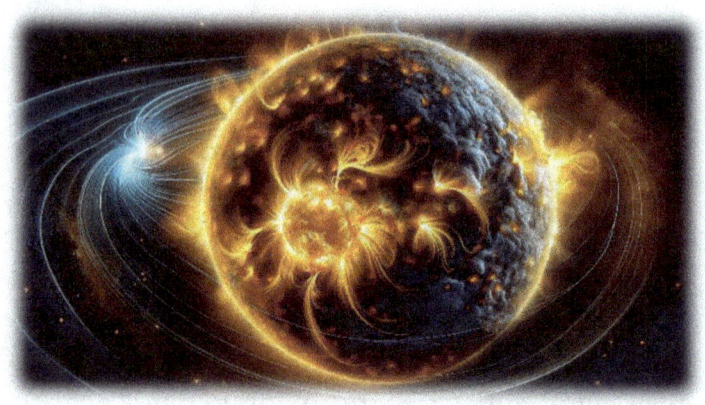

Geomagnetic storms result from the interaction between solar wind, carrying charged particles from CMEs, and Earth's magnetic field. These interactions can induce electric currents in the atmosphere and on the ground, affecting both natural and man-made systems. For humans, the primary concern lies in how these electromagnetic fluctuations can influence physiological and biochemical processes.

Central to this discussion are the effects on melatonin and serotonin, two critical hormones involved in regulating sleep, mood, and overall mental health. Melatonin, produced by the pineal gland in the brain, regulates the sleep-wake cycle and is influenced by light exposure. Serotonin, a neurotransmitter, plays a key role in mood regulation, appetite, and circadian rhythms. Disruptions in the levels of these hormones can lead to sleep disorders, depression, anxiety, and other health issues.

Studies have suggested that geomagnetic activity can alter melatonin production. For instance, some research indicates that melatonin levels decrease during periods of high geomagnetic activity, potentially disrupting sleep patterns and circadian rhythms. This effect is thought to be due to the interaction of geomagnetic fields with the human body's electromagnetic field, influencing the biochemical pathways involved in hormone production and regulation.

Similarly, serotonin levels may be affected by geomagnetic storms. There is evidence to suggest that increased geomagnetic activity correlates with higher incidences of mood disturbances, including depression and anxiety.

The mechanisms behind this are not fully understood, but it is hypothesized that geomagnetic fluctuations could impact serotonin metabolism or the neural pathways associated with mood regulation.

Beyond hormonal effects, there are other physiological impacts to consider. For example, cardiovascular health appears to be sensitive to geomagnetic activity. Some studies have shown a higher incidence of heart attacks and strokes during geomagnetic storms, suggesting that these events may influence blood clotting mechanisms or heart rate variability. Additionally, there is ongoing research into the neurological impacts, with some findings indicating changes in brain wave patterns and cognitive function during periods of high geomagnetic activity.

The radiation associated with solar flares and CMEs also poses risks, particularly for astronauts and high-altitude pilots. Increased exposure to solar radiation during intense solar storms can lead to DNA damage, increased cancer risk, and other health issues. While the Earth's atmosphere provides substantial protection against these effects for people on the ground, those in aviation or space exploration face greater risks.

This book aims to explore these fascinating interactions in detail. We will delve into the science behind solar activity and geomagnetic storms, examining their mechanisms and how they affect both technology and biology. We will review the current state of research on the physiological and biochemical impacts, focusing on melatonin and serotonin, cardiovascular health, and neurological effects. Through case studies and analysis of available data, we will highlight significant findings and identify areas where further research is needed.

Understanding the potential health effects of CMEs and solar flares is not only of scientific interest but also of practical importance. As we become increasingly dependent on technology vulnerable to solar activity, and as human space exploration advances, comprehending and mitigating these impacts will be crucial. By bringing together knowledge from various scientific disciplines, this book seeks to provide a comprehensive overview of this emerging field, offering insights and guidance for researchers, healthcare professionals, and anyone interested in the intersection of space weather and human health.

In the chapters that follow, we will embark on a journey through the cosmos and into the human body, exploring the powerful and sometimes surprising ways in which the sun's activity can influence our lives.

3 GEOMAGNETIC STORMS AND THEIR EFFECTS ON EARTH

The interaction between the sun's activity and Earth's magnetic field gives rise to geomagnetic storms—powerful disturbances that can have significant impacts on both natural and human-made systems. Understanding the mechanisms of geomagnetic storms and their wide-ranging effects is crucial for comprehending the full scope of solar activity's influence on our planet.

What are Geomagnetic Storms?

Geomagnetic storms occur when bursts of solar wind, typically from Coronal Mass Ejections (CMEs) or high-speed solar wind streams, interact with Earth's magnetosphere. These storms are characterized by rapid and intense variations in the Earth's magnetic field.

The primary components of a geomagnetic storm include:
- Initial Phase: A sudden increase in the Earth's magnetic field strength caused by the arrival of the shock wave from a CME.
- Main Phase: A period of significant disturbance in the magnetic field, usually lasting several hours to days, marked by a decrease in the geomagnetic field intensity.
- Recovery Phase: The magnetic field gradually returns to its normal state, which can take several days.

Geomagnetic storms are measured using the Kp index, a scale from 0 to 9 that quantifies the magnitude of geomagnetic activity. A Kp index of 5 or higher indicates a geomagnetic storm.

Causes of Geomagnetic Storms

The primary causes of geomagnetic storms are CMEs and solar wind streams from coronal holes:
- CMEs: These massive bursts of solar wind and magnetic fields can significantly disturb the Earth's magnetosphere upon impact.
- Coronal Holes: These are areas where the sun's corona is darker and colder, with open magnetic

field lines that allow high-speed solar wind to escape. When these streams reach Earth, they can enhance geomagnetic activity.

Interaction with the Magnetosphere

When the charged particles from solar wind or CMEs reach Earth, they compress the magnetosphere on the side facing the sun and create a long tail on the opposite side. This interaction causes energy to be transferred from the solar wind into the Earth's magnetosphere, leading to the following phenomena:

- Magnetospheric Convection: The circulation of plasma within the magnetosphere, driven by the interaction with the solar wind.
- Ring Current: A current of charged particles that encircles the Earth, which can intensify during geomagnetic storms and cause further disturbances in the magnetic field.
- Auroras: The most visually stunning effect of geomagnetic storms, auroras (Northern and Southern Lights) are caused by charged particles colliding with atmospheric gases, resulting in glowing light displays in polar regions.

Effects on Technology and Infrastructure

Geomagnetic storms can have profound impacts

on various technological systems:

- Power Grids: Geomagnetic storms induce electric currents in power lines, known as Geomagnetically Induced Currents (GICs). These currents can overload transformers and other components of the power grid, leading to voltage instability, equipment damage, and blackouts. The 1989 geomagnetic storm that caused a nine-hour blackout in Quebec, Canada, is a notable example of such an impact.

- Satellites and Spacecraft: Increased radiation and charged particle flux during geomagnetic storms can damage satellite electronics, affect satellite orbits due to atmospheric drag, and disrupt communication signals. Satellites in low Earth orbit are particularly vulnerable to these effects.

- Aviation: Geomagnetic storms pose risks to aviation by disrupting high-frequency radio communications, affecting GPS accuracy, and exposing high-altitude flights to increased radiation levels. Airlines may need to reroute polar flights to avoid communication blackouts and excessive radiation exposure.

- Communication Systems: High-frequency radio communications, which rely on the ionosphere, can be severely disrupted during geomagnetic storms. This affects military operations, emergency services, and transcontinental aviation, which rely on these communication systems.

- Oil and Gas Pipelines: Geomagnetically induced currents can also flow through pipelines, increasing corrosion rates and potentially leading to leaks and failures. Monitoring and mitigating these effects are crucial for maintaining pipeline integrity.

Natural Effects and Phenomena

Beyond technological impacts, geomagnetic storms also induce various natural phenomena:

- Auroras: As mentioned, auroras are the result of charged particles colliding with gases in Earth's atmosphere. During strong geomagnetic storms, auroras can be seen at much lower latitudes than usual, providing spectacular displays far from the polar regions.

- Animal Navigation: Many animals, including birds, sea turtles, and even some insects, rely on Earth's magnetic field for navigation. Geomagnetic storms can disrupt these natural navigation systems, leading to confusion and disorientation in migratory patterns.

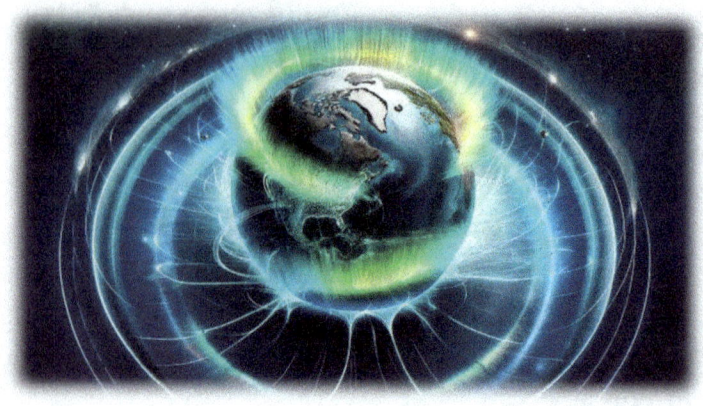

Geomagnetic Storms and Human Health

While the direct effects of geomagnetic storms on human health are less immediately apparent than their technological impacts, there is growing evidence suggesting that these storms can influence human physiology and well-being. These potential health effects are explored in greater detail in subsequent chapters, particularly focusing on cardiovascular health, neurological impacts, and hormone regulation.

Historical Context of Geomagnetic Storms

Several significant geomagnetic storms have been recorded throughout history, providing valuable insights into their potential impacts:

- The Carrington Event (1859): The largest geomagnetic storm on record, this event caused widespread auroras and disrupted telegraph systems across Europe and North America. Named after the British astronomer Richard Carrington, who observed the associated solar flare, the Carrington Event serves as a benchmark for understanding the potential severity of geomagnetic storms.

- The 1989 Quebec Blackout: This storm caused a nine-hour blackout in Quebec, Canada, by inducing electric currents in power lines that overloaded transformers. The event highlighted the vulnerability of modern power grids to geomagnetic storms.

- The Halloween Storms (2003): A series of strong geomagnetic storms in late October 2003 disrupted satellite communications, caused power outages in Sweden, and produced auroras visible as far south as Texas. These storms demonstrated the wide-ranging impacts of solar activity on contemporary technology.

This chapter has provided an overview of geomagnetic storms, their causes, and their effects on both technology and natural systems. By understanding the mechanisms behind these storms and their historical impacts, we can better appreciate the potential risks and challenges they pose to modern society. As we move forward, we will delve deeper into the specific ways geomagnetic storms influence human health, exploring the intricate connections between solar activity and our own physiological and biochemical processes.

4 GEOMAGNETIC STORMS AND EARTH'S CLIMATE

The interplay between geomagnetic storms and Earth's climate is a topic of growing interest and debate within the scientific community. While the direct effects of solar activity on technology and human health are well-documented, the potential connections between geomagnetic storms and climate patterns remain less clear. This chapter delves into the possible mechanisms by which solar activity could influence climate, reviews the evidence from historical and contemporary studies, and discusses the ongoing scientific debates and future research directions.

The Sun's Influence on Earth's Climate

The sun is the primary driver of Earth's climate system. Solar radiation provides the energy that powers atmospheric circulation, ocean currents, and weather patterns. Variations in solar output can, therefore, have significant effects on climate. These variations include changes in the sun's luminosity, the 11-year solar cycle, and sporadic events such as solar flares and Coronal Mass Ejections (CMEs).

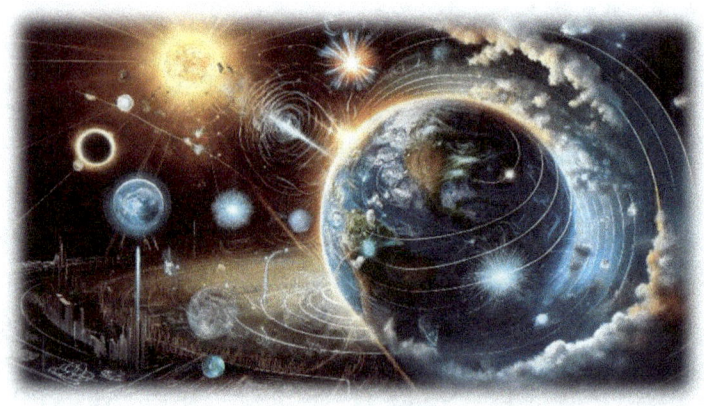

Solar Cycles and Climate Variability

The most well-known solar cycle is the approximately 11-year cycle of sunspot activity, which corresponds to fluctuations in solar radiation. During periods of high sunspot activity (solar maximum), the sun emits slightly more radiation. Conversely, during periods of low sunspot activity (solar minimum), solar radiation decreases. These changes in solar output can influence Earth's climate, though the effects are generally small compared to other factors such as greenhouse gas concentrations.

Historical records suggest correlations between solar cycles and climate variability. For example, the Maunder Minimum (1645-1715), a period of unusually low sunspot activity, coincided with the "Little Ice Age," a time of cooler temperatures in Europe and North America. However, establishing a direct causal relationship is challenging due to the multitude of factors influencing climate.

Geomagnetic Storms and Atmospheric Chemistry

Geomagnetic storms, caused by the interaction of CMEs and high-speed solar wind streams with Earth's magnetosphere, can influence atmospheric chemistry. These storms can enhance the production of nitric oxide and other reactive nitrogen species in the upper atmosphere. These reactive species can deplete ozone in the stratosphere, potentially affecting temperature and atmospheric circulation patterns.

1. Ozone Depletion: Enhanced production of nitric oxide during geomagnetic storms can lead to temporary ozone depletion in the stratosphere. Ozone plays a critical role in absorbing ultraviolet (UV) radiation from the sun, and changes in ozone concentrations can influence stratospheric temperatures and dynamics.

2. Atmospheric Circulation: Changes in stratospheric ozone can alter atmospheric circulation patterns. For example, ozone depletion can lead to cooling in the stratosphere, which may affect the jet stream and other large-scale atmospheric circulation features.

Cosmic Rays and Cloud Formation

Another proposed mechanism by which solar activity could influence climate involves cosmic rays. Galactic cosmic rays are high-energy particles from outside the solar system that continuously bombard Earth. The intensity of cosmic rays reaching Earth's atmosphere is modulated by the sun's magnetic field, which is stronger during periods of high solar activity and weaker during solar minimums.

1. Cloud Condensation Nuclei: Cosmic rays can

ionize molecules in the atmosphere, leading to the formation of aerosols that can act as cloud condensation nuclei (CCN). An increase in CCN can enhance cloud formation, which can affect Earth's radiative balance by reflecting more sunlight back into space (albedo effect).

2. Cloud Cover and Climate: Changes in cloud cover can influence climate by altering the Earth's albedo and the greenhouse effect. Increased cloud cover can lead to cooling by reflecting more sunlight, while certain types of clouds can contribute to warming by trapping infrared radiation.

Evidence from Historical and Contemporary Studies

Research into the connections between geomagnetic storms, solar activity, and climate involves a combination of historical data analysis, climate modeling, and empirical observations.

Historical Climate Records

1. Little Ice Age and Maunder Minimum: The Maunder Minimum, a period of low sunspot activity from 1645 to 1715, coincided with the coldest part of the Little Ice Age. During this

time, Europe and North America experienced cooler temperatures, harsher winters, and shorter growing seasons. While this correlation suggests a link between low solar activity and cooler climate, it is important to note that other factors, such as volcanic activity, also played a significant role.

2. Medieval Warm Period: Conversely, the Medieval Warm Period (approx. 950-1250 AD) was characterized by relatively warm temperatures and high solar activity. This period saw flourishing civilizations and agricultural expansion in regions such as Europe and North America. Again, while solar activity may have contributed to these climatic conditions, other factors must be considered.

Contemporary Observations and Models

1. Satellite Data: Modern satellite observations provide detailed measurements of solar radiation, cosmic rays, and atmospheric conditions. These data have been used to investigate potential links between solar activity and climate. For example, studies have examined correlations between solar cycles and variations in cloud cover, temperature, and atmospheric circulation.

2. Climate Models: Climate models incorporating solar variability and cosmic ray effects have been developed to simulate potential impacts on climate. These models suggest that while solar activity can influence climate, the effects are generally smaller compared to other anthropogenic factors, such as greenhouse gas emissions.

3. Empirical Studies: Empirical studies have explored the effects of specific geomagnetic storms on atmospheric conditions. For example, research has shown temporary changes in stratospheric ozone concentrations and atmospheric circulation patterns following major geomagnetic storms. These studies provide valuable insights but also highlight the complexity of isolating the impacts of solar activity from other climatic factors.

Ongoing Scientific Debates

The potential connections between geomagnetic storms, solar activity, and climate remain a topic of active research and debate. Key areas of contention include:

1. Magnitude of Effects: While there is evidence that solar activity can influence climate, the magnitude of these effects relative to other

factors, such as greenhouse gases, is debated. Many scientists argue that the impact of solar variability is relatively small in the context of contemporary climate change driven by human activities.

2. Mechanistic Pathways: The specific mechanisms by which solar activity influences climate are complex and not fully understood. Further research is needed to elucidate the pathways through which geomagnetic storms and cosmic rays may affect atmospheric chemistry, cloud formation, and climate.

3. Attribution Challenges: Separating the effects of solar activity from other climatic influences is challenging. Climate is influenced by a multitude of factors, including volcanic activity, ocean currents, and anthropogenic emissions. Disentangling these influences requires sophisticated modeling and long-term data analysis.

Future Research Directions

To advance our understanding of the connections between geomagnetic storms and climate, several research directions are recommended:

1. Long-Term Data Collection: Continued collection and analysis of long-term climate and solar activity data are essential for identifying patterns and correlations. This includes historical climate records, satellite observations, and atmospheric measurements.

2. Integrated Climate Models: Developing and refining climate models that incorporate solar variability, cosmic ray effects, and other relevant factors will enhance our ability to simulate and predict the impacts of solar activity on climate.

3. Mechanistic Studies: Research focused on the specific mechanisms by which solar activity influences atmospheric chemistry and cloud formation will provide deeper insights into the pathways linking geomagnetic storms and climate.

4. Interdisciplinary Collaboration: Collaboration between solar physicists, atmospheric scientists, climatologists, and other researchers is crucial for advancing our understanding of this complex topic. Interdisciplinary approaches can integrate diverse perspectives and methodologies.

5. Public Communication: Effective communication of scientific findings to policymakers and the public is important for

informed decision-making. This includes conveying the uncertainties and complexities of the science while highlighting the potential implications for climate and environmental policy.

The exploration of possible connections between geomagnetic storms and climate reveals a fascinating and complex interplay between solar activity and Earth's climate system. While the direct impacts of geomagnetic storms on technology and human health are well-established, their potential influence on climate remains an area of active investigation and debate.

Understanding these connections requires a multidisciplinary approach that integrates historical data, contemporary observations, and sophisticated climate models. By advancing our knowledge of the mechanisms and pathways linking solar activity and climate, we can better anticipate and mitigate the impacts of geomagnetic storms on our planet.

As we continue to explore the dynamic relationship between the sun and Earth, it is essential to recognize the broader implications for climate science, environmental policy, and societal resilience. The insights gained from this research will contribute to our ability to navigate the challenges and opportunities presented by our ever-changing sun, ensuring a sustainable and resilient future for all.

5 HUMAN PHYSIOLOGY AND BIOCHEMISTRY

The interaction between solar activity and human health is a complex and intriguing field of study. While the Earth's atmosphere and magnetic field provide substantial protection against the direct impacts of solar radiation and charged particles, geomagnetic storms induced by solar flares and Coronal Mass Ejections (CMEs) can still affect human physiology and biochemistry. This chapter delves into the fundamental aspects of human physiology that may be influenced by geomagnetic activity, focusing on the cardiovascular system, neurological effects, and hormone regulation, particularly melatonin and serotonin.

Human Physiology: An Overview

Human physiology encompasses the functions and mechanisms operating within the human body. It involves various systems, including the cardiovascular, nervous, endocrine, and immune systems, all of which can potentially be influenced by external environmental factors such as geomagnetic storms. Understanding these physiological systems is essential for exploring how geomagnetic activity might impact human health.

Cardiovascular System

The cardiovascular system, consisting of the heart, blood vessels, and blood, is crucial for maintaining life by delivering oxygen and nutrients to tissues and removing waste products. Geomagnetic storms have been associated with several cardiovascular effects:

- Heart Rate Variability (HRV): HRV refers to the variation in time between each heartbeat, which is an indicator of autonomic nervous system function and cardiovascular health. Studies have shown that geomagnetic storms can influence HRV, potentially leading to increased stress on the cardiovascular system.

- Blood Pressure and Circulation: Some research suggests that geomagnetic activity may affect blood pressure and circulation. For instance, increased geomagnetic activity has been linked to higher blood pressure and changes in blood flow, possibly due to the body's response to electromagnetic fluctuations.

- Cardiovascular Events: Epidemiological studies have reported correlations between geomagnetic storms and the incidence of heart attacks and strokes. The underlying mechanisms are not fully understood, but it is hypothesized that geomagnetic activity may influence blood clotting and inflammatory processes, contributing to cardiovascular events.

Neurological Effects

The nervous system, including the brain, spinal cord, and peripheral nerves, controls and coordinates bodily functions. Geomagnetic storms can potentially influence neurological health in various ways:

- Brain Activity and Cognitive Function: Geomagnetic activity can affect brain wave patterns and cognitive function. Some studies have observed changes in electroencephalogram (EEG) readings during geomagnetic storms, suggesting that the brain's electrical activity can be influenced by external electromagnetic fields.

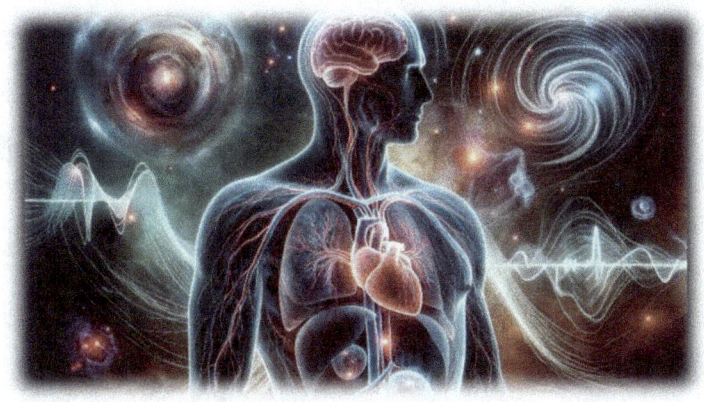

- Mood and Mental Health: There is evidence to suggest that geomagnetic storms can impact mood and mental health. Increased geomagnetic activity has been associated with higher incidences of mood disorders, such as depression and anxiety. The exact mechanisms remain unclear, but it is believed that geomagnetic fluctuations may affect neurotransmitter levels and brain function.

- Sleep Patterns: Geomagnetic activity can also disrupt sleep patterns. Melatonin, a hormone that regulates sleep, may be influenced by geomagnetic storms, leading to sleep disturbances. Poor sleep quality and altered sleep patterns can have cascading effects on overall health and well-being.

Hormone Regulation: Melatonin and Serotonin

Melatonin and serotonin are two critical hormones involved in regulating sleep, mood, and other physiological processes. Understanding their roles and how geomagnetic activity might influence their levels is key to exploring the broader health impacts of solar activity.

- Melatonin: Produced by the pineal gland in response to darkness, melatonin regulates the sleep-wake cycle and other circadian rhythms. It is known as the "sleep hormone" because it helps signal to the body that it is time to sleep. Research indicates that geomagnetic storms can reduce melatonin production, likely due to the interaction between geomagnetic fields and the body's electromagnetic environment. Reduced melatonin levels can lead to sleep disturbances, affecting overall health.

- Serotonin: Serotonin is a neurotransmitter that plays a crucial role in mood regulation, appetite, and sleep. It is often referred to as the "feel-good" hormone because of its influence on well-being and happiness. Geomagnetic storms may impact serotonin levels, potentially leading to mood disturbances and mental health issues. The exact pathways through which geomagnetic activity influences serotonin are not well understood, but changes in brain electrical activity and neurotransmitter synthesis are possible factors.

Oxidative Stress and Inflammation

Geomagnetic activity can also induce oxidative stress and inflammation in the body, which are underlying factors in many chronic diseases:

- Oxidative Stress: Exposure to increased levels of solar radiation and geomagnetic fluctuations can lead to the production of reactive oxygen species (ROS), which cause oxidative damage to cells and tissues. This oxidative stress can affect various organs and systems, contributing to aging and disease.

- Inflammatory Response: Geomagnetic storms may trigger inflammatory responses in the body. Chronic inflammation is linked to a range of health conditions, including cardiovascular disease, neurodegenerative disorders, and autoimmune diseases. Understanding how geomagnetic activity influences inflammation can provide insights into its broader health impacts.

Case Studies and Epidemiological Research

Several case studies and epidemiological studies have explored the potential health impacts of geomagnetic storms:

- Case Study: The 1989 Quebec Blackout: During the 1989 geomagnetic storm that caused a blackout in Quebec, researchers observed an increase in hospital admissions for cardiovascular issues. This case highlights the potential for geomagnetic storms to exacerbate pre-existing health conditions.

- Epidemiological Studies: Various studies have examined correlations between geomagnetic activity and health outcomes. For example, some research has found increased incidences of heart attacks, strokes, and psychiatric hospital admissions during periods of high geomagnetic activity. While these studies suggest potential links, more research is needed to establish causality and understand the underlying mechanisms.

This chapter has explored the fundamental aspects of human physiology and biochemistry that may be influenced by geomagnetic storms.

The cardiovascular system, neurological health, and hormone regulation are particularly susceptible to these external environmental factors. Understanding the complex interactions between geomagnetic activity and human health is crucial for developing strategies to mitigate potential risks and enhance our resilience to solar-induced disturbances.

As we move forward, the subsequent chapters will delve deeper into specific health impacts, reviewing scientific studies and case examples to provide a comprehensive understanding of this emerging field. By examining the intricate connections between solar activity and our own biological systems, we aim to shed light on the profound ways in which the cosmos influences our lives.

6 CARDIOVASCULAR AND NEUROLOGICAL EFFECTS

The potential impact of geomagnetic storms on human health extends to critical physiological systems, notably the cardiovascular and neurological systems. Understanding how these systems respond to geomagnetic disturbances can help in identifying vulnerable populations and developing preventive strategies. This chapter explores the effects of geomagnetic storms on cardiovascular health, heart rate variability, blood pressure, and the nervous system, including cognitive function, mood, and mental health.

Cardiovascular Health

The cardiovascular system is vital for sustaining

life, as it is responsible for delivering oxygen and nutrients to tissues and removing waste products. Research has suggested that geomagnetic storms can influence cardiovascular health in several ways:

Heart Rate Variability (HRV)

Heart rate variability (HRV) is the variation in the time interval between consecutive heartbeats. It is a measure of autonomic nervous system function and an indicator of cardiovascular health and stress levels. High HRV generally indicates a healthy heart with good autonomic function, while low HRV is associated with stress, fatigue, and increased risk of cardiovascular disease.

- Impact of Geomagnetic Storms on HRV: Studies have shown that geomagnetic storms can affect HRV, often leading to reduced variability. This suggests increased stress on the cardiovascular system during periods of high geomagnetic activity. Reduced HRV during geomagnetic storms may be due to increased sympathetic nervous system activity (the "fight or flight" response) and reduced parasympathetic activity (the "rest and digest" response).

Blood Pressure and Circulation

Geomagnetic storms may also influence blood pressure and circulation, though the mechanisms are not entirely clear:

- Blood Pressure Changes: Some studies have reported changes in blood pressure during geomagnetic storms. For example, increased geomagnetic activity has been associated with higher blood pressure levels. This effect could be mediated by stress responses and changes in autonomic nervous system function.

- Circulatory Effects: Geomagnetic disturbances may affect blood flow and circulation. There is evidence to suggest that geomagnetic activity can alter blood viscosity and clotting mechanisms, potentially increasing the risk of thrombotic events such as heart attacks and strokes.

Cardiovascular Events

Epidemiological research has explored the correlation between geomagnetic storms and cardiovascular events:

- Heart Attacks and Strokes: Several studies have found an increased incidence of heart attacks and strokes during periods of high geomagnetic activity. For instance, a study conducted during the 1989 geomagnetic storm that caused the Quebec blackout reported a significant rise in hospital admissions for cardiovascular issues. The proposed mechanisms include changes in blood clotting, increased oxidative stress, and inflammatory responses triggered by geomagnetic disturbances.

Neurological Effects

The nervous system, comprising the brain, spinal cord, and peripheral nerves, is highly sensitive to external electromagnetic fields. Geomagnetic storms can influence brain function, cognitive abilities, and mental health.

Brain Activity and Cognitive Function

- EEG Changes: Electroencephalogram (EEG) studies have shown that geomagnetic storms can alter brain wave patterns. These changes in electrical activity may affect cognitive functions such as attention, memory, and executive function. Some research suggests that individuals may experience reduced cognitive performance and increased mental fatigue during geomagnetic storms.

- Cognitive Impairment: There is evidence that

geomagnetic activity can impair cognitive function, particularly in tasks requiring sustained attention and mental effort. This impairment could be related to disruptions in brain electrical activity and neurotransmitter levels.

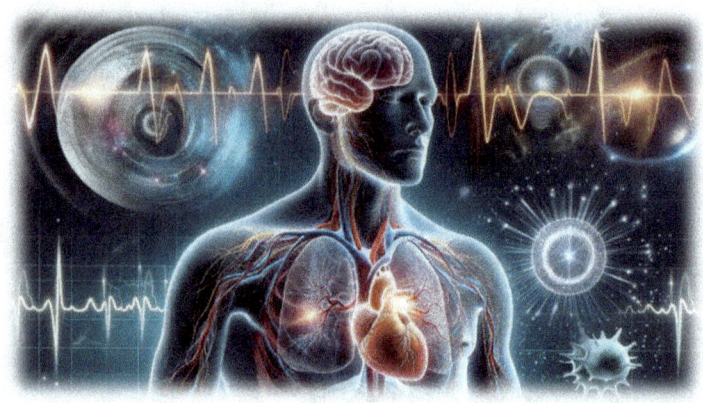

Mood and Mental Health

Geomagnetic storms have been associated with mood disturbances and mental health issues:

- Mood Disorders: Increased geomagnetic activity has been linked to higher incidences of mood disorders such as depression and anxiety. The exact mechanisms are not well understood, but it is hypothesized that geomagnetic fluctuations may affect serotonin levels and other neurotransmitters involved in mood regulation.

- Psychiatric Hospital Admissions: Some epidemiological studies have observed a rise in psychiatric hospital admissions during geomagnetic storms. This correlation suggests that geomagnetic activity may exacerbate pre-existing mental health conditions or trigger new episodes of psychiatric disorders.

Sleep Patterns

Sleep quality and patterns can be influenced by geomagnetic activity, primarily through its effects on melatonin production:

- Melatonin Disruption: Melatonin, a hormone produced by the pineal gland, regulates sleep-wake cycles. Geomagnetic storms can reduce melatonin levels, leading to sleep disturbances such as insomnia and poor sleep quality. Disrupted sleep can have cascading effects on overall health, contributing to fatigue, cognitive impairment, and mood disturbances.

Case Studies and Epidemiological Evidence

Several case studies and epidemiological investigations provide insights into the cardiovascular and neurological impacts of geomagnetic storms:

- The 1989 Quebec Blackout: During this major geomagnetic storm, researchers observed an increase in hospital admissions for both cardiovascular and neurological issues. This event highlighted the potential for geomagnetic storms to affect human health on a large scale.

- Epidemiological Correlations: Numerous studies have examined the links between geomagnetic activity and health outcomes. For example, a study published in the *American Journal of Epidemiology* reported a significant association between high geomagnetic activity and increased mortality due to cardiovascular causes. Other research has found correlations between geomagnetic storms and psychiatric hospital admissions, providing further evidence of the health impacts of geomagnetic disturbances.

Mechanisms and Hypotheses

The exact mechanisms through which geomagnetic storms influence cardiovascular and neurological health are not fully understood, but several hypotheses have been proposed:

- Electromagnetic Field Interactions: Geomagnetic storms generate fluctuations in the

Earth's electromagnetic field, which may interact with the human body's own electromagnetic fields. These interactions could affect cellular and molecular processes, influencing heart rate variability, blood pressure, and brain activity.

- Oxidative Stress and Inflammation: Geomagnetic activity may induce oxidative stress and inflammatory responses in the body. Increased levels of reactive oxygen species (ROS) and inflammatory markers can damage cells and tissues, contributing to cardiovascular and neurological conditions.

- Autonomic Nervous System: The autonomic nervous system, which regulates involuntary bodily functions, may be affected by geomagnetic fluctuations. Changes in autonomic balance could influence heart rate, blood pressure, and stress responses, impacting overall cardiovascular and neurological health.

This chapter has explored the cardiovascular and neurological effects of geomagnetic storms, highlighting the potential health risks associated with solar activity. Geomagnetic storms can influence heart rate variability, blood pressure, cognitive function, mood, and sleep patterns, potentially leading to significant health impacts. Understanding these effects and the underlying mechanisms is crucial for identifying vulnerable populations and developing strategies to mitigate the risks.

As we continue to explore the connections between solar activity and human health, the subsequent chapters will delve into hormonal effects, oxidative stress, and the broader implications for public health. By integrating insights from various scientific disciplines, we aim to provide a comprehensive understanding of the complex interactions between the cosmos and our own biological systems.

7 HORMONAL EFFECTS: MELATONIN AND SEROTONIN

The potential influence of geomagnetic storms on human health extends to the regulation of critical hormones, particularly melatonin and serotonin. These hormones play essential roles in maintaining circadian rhythms, mood, and overall mental health. Understanding how geomagnetic activity might disrupt the balance of these hormones provides deeper insights into the broader physiological impacts of solar activity on human well-being.

Melatonin: The Sleep Hormone

Melatonin is a hormone produced by the pineal gland in the brain in response to darkness. It is a key regulator of the sleep-wake cycle and other circadian rhythms. Melatonin's primary function is to signal to the body that it is time to sleep, promoting restful and restorative sleep.

Production and Regulation

Melatonin production follows a daily cycle, with levels rising in the evening as it gets dark and peaking during the night. Light exposure, especially blue light, inhibits melatonin synthesis, while darkness stimulates its production. This regulatory mechanism helps synchronize the body's internal clock with the external environment.

Geomagnetic Activity and Melatonin

Research has suggested that geomagnetic storms can affect melatonin production and secretion. Several studies have found correlations between increased geomagnetic activity and reduced melatonin levels. The hypothesized mechanisms for this effect include:

- Electromagnetic Interference: Geomagnetic storms generate fluctuations in the Earth's magnetic field, which can interact with the human body's electromagnetic fields. These interactions might disrupt the pineal gland's ability to produce melatonin.

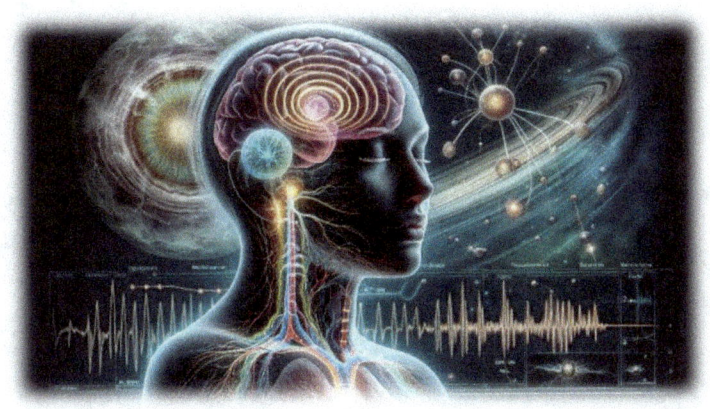

- Oxidative Stress: Geomagnetic storms can induce oxidative stress, leading to the production of reactive oxygen species (ROS). Oxidative stress can affect cellular functions, including hormone synthesis. Increased ROS levels may interfere with melatonin production pathways.

Health Implications of Melatonin Disruption

Reduced melatonin levels due to geomagnetic activity can have several health consequences:

- Sleep Disorders: Lower melatonin levels can lead to sleep disturbances such as insomnia, poor sleep quality, and disrupted sleep patterns. Chronic sleep deprivation is associated with numerous health issues, including weakened immune function, impaired cognitive performance, and increased risk of chronic diseases.

- Circadian Rhythm Disruption: Disrupted melatonin production can desynchronize the body's internal clock, affecting not only sleep but also other physiological processes governed by circadian rhythms, such as hormone release, metabolism, and mood regulation.

Serotonin: The Mood Stabilizer

Serotonin is a neurotransmitter that plays a crucial role in regulating mood, appetite, sleep, and other functions. It is often referred to as the "feel-good" hormone because of its significant influence on mood and emotional well-being.

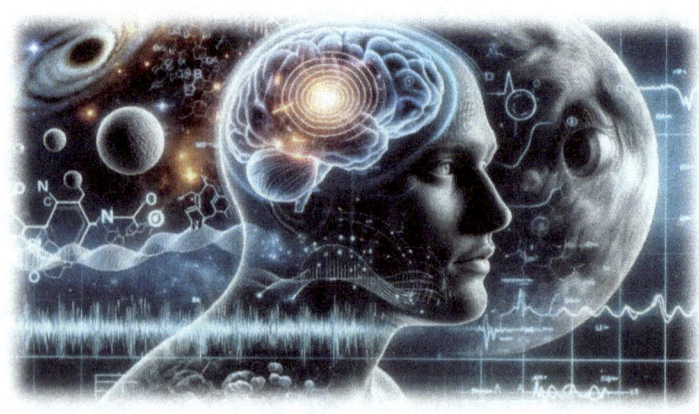

Production and Regulation

Serotonin is primarily produced in the gastrointestinal tract, with a smaller amount synthesized in the brain. Its production is influenced by various factors, including light exposure, diet, and physical activity. Serotonin levels typically follow a diurnal pattern, with higher levels during the day and lower levels at night.

Geomagnetic Activity and Serotonin

While research on the direct effects of geomagnetic activity on serotonin is less extensive than that on melatonin, there is evidence to suggest that geomagnetic storms may influence serotonin levels and metabolism. Possible mechanisms include:

- Neurotransmitter Regulation: Geomagnetic storms may affect the brain's electrical activity, potentially altering neurotransmitter synthesis and release. Changes in brain wave patterns during geomagnetic storms could influence serotonin pathways.

- Stress Response: Geomagnetic activity can

induce physiological stress, which might impact serotonin production and metabolism. The body's response to stress involves various hormonal changes, including alterations in serotonin levels.

Health Implications of Serotonin Disruption

Changes in serotonin levels due to geomagnetic activity can impact mental health and mood:

- Mood Disorders: Altered serotonin levels are associated with mood disorders such as depression and anxiety. Increased geomagnetic activity has been linked to higher incidences of these conditions, possibly due to disruptions in serotonin regulation.

- Cognitive Function: Serotonin plays a role in cognitive processes such as memory, learning, and attention. Disruptions in serotonin levels during geomagnetic storms could impair cognitive function and increase the risk of mental fatigue and cognitive decline.

Combined Effects on Health

The combined effects of disrupted melatonin and serotonin levels due to geomagnetic activity can lead to a range of health issues:

- Sleep and Mood Interactions: Melatonin and serotonin are interconnected in regulating sleep and mood. Disruptions in melatonin can affect serotonin levels and vice versa, creating a feedback loop that exacerbates sleep disorders and mood disturbances.

- Chronic Health Conditions: Long-term disruptions in melatonin and serotonin can contribute to the development of chronic health conditions, including cardiovascular disease, mental health disorders, and metabolic syndrome.

Case Studies and Epidemiological Evidence

Several studies and case examples provide insights into the hormonal effects of geomagnetic storms:

- Epidemiological Studies: Research has found correlations between periods of high geomagnetic activity and increased rates of mood disorders, sleep disturbances, and hospital admissions for psychiatric conditions. These studies suggest a link between geomagnetic storms and disruptions in melatonin and serotonin regulation.

- Case Studies: Individual case studies have reported exacerbations of mood disorders and sleep problems during geomagnetic storms. For instance, patients with pre-existing mental health conditions may experience worsening symptoms during periods of high geomagnetic activity.

Mechanisms and Hypotheses

Understanding the precise mechanisms through which geomagnetic storms influence melatonin and serotonin is an ongoing area of research. Several hypotheses have been proposed:

- Electromagnetic Field Interactions: Geomagnetic fluctuations may interfere with the body's electromagnetic environment, affecting the pineal gland and brain regions involved in hormone synthesis.

- Oxidative Stress: Increased oxidative stress during geomagnetic storms can impact cellular functions and hormone production pathways.

- Autonomic Nervous System: Geomagnetic activity may influence the autonomic nervous system, which regulates involuntary bodily functions, including hormone secretion.

This chapter has explored the effects of geomagnetic storms on the regulation of melatonin and serotonin, two critical hormones involved in sleep and mood regulation. Geomagnetic activity can disrupt the production and balance of these hormones, leading to sleep disorders, mood disturbances, and broader health implications. Understanding these effects and the underlying mechanisms is essential for developing strategies to mitigate the health risks associated with solar activity.

As we continue to delve into the broader implications of solar activity on human health, the subsequent chapters will examine oxidative stress, immune responses, and potential protective measures. By integrating insights from various scientific disciplines, we aim to provide a comprehensive understanding of the complex interactions between solar activity and our biological systems.

Aeron P. White

8 MENTAL HEALTH AND SPACE WEATHER

The relationship between space weather, particularly geomagnetic storms, and mental health is an emerging area of research that explores how fluctuations in the Earth's magnetic field can influence psychological well-being. While the physiological impacts of geomagnetic storms are increasingly documented, their potential psychological effects are less well understood. This chapter delves into the evidence linking geomagnetic activity with mental health outcomes, examines potential mechanisms, and discusses the implications for public health and future research.

Overview of Space Weather

Space weather refers to the conditions in space influenced by the sun and its activity, including solar flares, Coronal Mass Ejections (CMEs), and the solar wind. These phenomena can disrupt Earth's magnetosphere, leading to geomagnetic storms. While space weather is known to affect technology and human physiology, its influence on mental health is a relatively new area of inquiry.

Evidence Linking Geomagnetic Activity to Mental Health

Numerous studies have suggested correlations between geomagnetic storms and various mental health issues, including mood disorders, cognitive impairments, and psychiatric hospital admissions.

Mood Disorders

1. Depression and Anxiety: Several studies have found an association between increased geomagnetic activity and higher rates of depression and anxiety. For example, research published in the *Journal of Affective Disorders* observed a significant correlation between geomagnetic storms and the incidence

of depressive episodes.

2. Seasonal Affective Disorder (SAD): There is some evidence to suggest that geomagnetic storms may exacerbate symptoms of Seasonal Affective Disorder (SAD), a type of depression that occurs at certain times of the year, typically in winter. The disruption of melatonin production during geomagnetic storms could be a contributing factor.

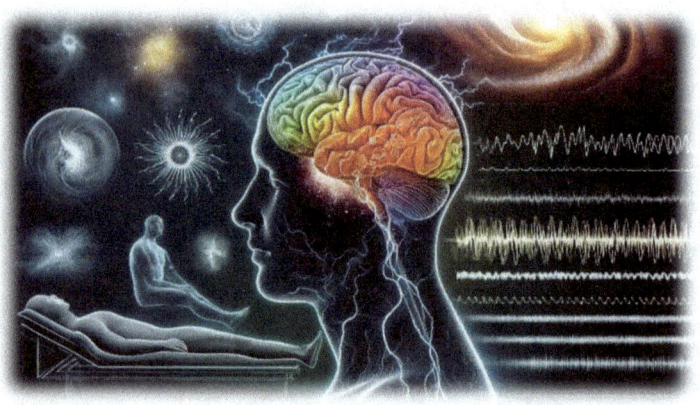

Cognitive Impairments

1. Attention and Memory: Geomagnetic activity has been linked to temporary impairments in cognitive functions such as attention and memory. Studies have shown changes in brain wave patterns during geomagnetic storms, which may affect cognitive

performance.

2. Mental Fatigue: Increased geomagnetic activity can lead to symptoms of mental fatigue and reduced cognitive efficiency. This may be due to the additional stress placed on the body and brain by fluctuations in the Earth's magnetic field.

Psychiatric Hospital Admissions

1. Increased Admissions: Some epidemiological studies have reported spikes in psychiatric hospital admissions during periods of high geomagnetic activity. For instance, research conducted in the UK and Russia found that hospital admissions for psychiatric conditions increased significantly during geomagnetic storms.

2. Exacerbation of Pre-existing Conditions: Geomagnetic storms may exacerbate symptoms in individuals with pre-existing psychiatric conditions, leading to higher rates of hospital admissions and more severe symptoms.

Potential Mechanisms

The mechanisms by which geomagnetic activity might influence mental health are complex and multifaceted. Several hypotheses have been proposed to explain these associations.

Electromagnetic Field Interactions

1. Brain Electromagnetic Activity: The human brain generates its own electromagnetic fields, which are essential for normal neurological function. Geomagnetic storms can cause fluctuations in the Earth's magnetic field that might interfere with the brain's electromagnetic activity, potentially disrupting cognitive and emotional processes.

2. Pineal Gland and Melatonin: The pineal gland, which produces melatonin, is sensitive to electromagnetic fields. Geomagnetic storms can disrupt melatonin production, leading to sleep disturbances and mood changes. Melatonin is crucial for regulating sleep-wake cycles and mood, and its disruption can have wide-ranging effects on mental health.

Oxidative Stress and Inflammation

1. Reactive Oxygen Species (ROS): Geomagnetic storms can increase the production of reactive oxygen species (ROS) in the body, leading to oxidative stress. Oxidative stress can

damage cells and tissues, including those in the brain, contributing to neurological and psychological disorders.

2. Inflammatory Response: Increased geomagnetic activity may trigger inflammatory responses in the body. Chronic inflammation is associated with various mental health conditions, including depression and anxiety. Understanding how geomagnetic storms influence inflammation could provide insights into their psychological impacts.

Autonomic Nervous System

1. Autonomic Dysregulation: Geomagnetic storms can affect the autonomic nervous system (ANS), which regulates involuntary physiological functions such as heart rate, digestion, and respiratory rate. Dysregulation of the ANS can lead to symptoms of anxiety and stress, contributing to mental health issues.

2. Heart Rate Variability (HRV): Changes in heart rate variability (HRV), a measure of autonomic function, have been observed during geomagnetic storms. Lower HRV is associated with increased stress and anxiety, suggesting a possible link between geomagnetic activity and psychological well-being.

Implications for Public Health

Understanding the potential psychological impacts of geomagnetic storms has important implications for public health. By recognizing the influence of space weather on mental health, healthcare providers and public health officials can develop strategies to mitigate these effects.

Monitoring and Forecasting

1. Space Weather Monitoring: Continuous monitoring of space weather conditions can provide valuable data for predicting periods of high geomagnetic activity. Early warning systems can help individuals and healthcare providers prepare for potential mental health impacts.

2. Mental Health Surveillance: Integrating space weather data with mental health surveillance systems can help identify patterns and correlations between geomagnetic activity and mental health outcomes. This information can guide public health interventions and resource allocation.

Public Awareness and Education

1. Educational Campaigns: Public education

campaigns can raise awareness about the potential psychological impacts of geomagnetic storms and promote strategies for coping with these effects. This includes providing information on sleep hygiene, stress management, and mental health resources.

2. Community Engagement: Engaging communities in discussions about space weather and mental health can enhance resilience. Community leaders, mental health organizations, and educational institutions can play a key role in disseminating information and supporting affected individuals.

Protective Measures

1. Stress Management Techniques: Encouraging the use of stress management techniques, such as mindfulness, meditation, and regular physical activity, can help individuals cope with the psychological impacts of geomagnetic storms.

2. Mental Health Support Services: Ensuring access to mental health support services during periods of high geomagnetic activity is crucial. This includes providing counseling, crisis intervention, and support groups for individuals experiencing mental health challenges.

Future Research Directions

Further research is needed to fully understand the psychological impacts of geomagnetic storms and develop effective interventions. Key areas for future research include:

1. Mechanistic Studies: Investigating the specific biological and physiological mechanisms by which geomagnetic activity influences mental health will provide deeper insights into this complex relationship.

2. Longitudinal Studies: Long-term studies tracking mental health outcomes in relation to geomagnetic activity can help identify chronic effects and inform prevention strategies.

3. Interdisciplinary Collaboration: Collaboration between space scientists, neuroscientists, psychologists, and public health experts is essential for advancing our understanding of the psychological impacts of space weather.

4. Intervention Development: Developing and testing interventions to mitigate the psychological effects of geomagnetic storms will be crucial for protecting mental health. This

includes exploring pharmacological, behavioral, and technological solutions.

The exploration of the psychological impacts of geomagnetic storms reveals a complex and intriguing interplay between space weather and mental health. While the evidence suggests that geomagnetic activity can influence mood, cognitive function, and psychiatric conditions, much remains to be understood about the underlying mechanisms and long-term effects.

By advancing research in this area and developing effective public health strategies, we can better anticipate and mitigate the psychological impacts of geomagnetic storms. As our understanding of space weather continues to grow, so too will our ability to protect and promote mental health in the face of these dynamic and powerful natural phenomena. The insights gained from this research will contribute to a more resilient and informed society, capable of navigating the challenges and opportunities presented by our ever-changing sun.

9 RADIATION EFFECTS

The sun's activity, particularly during solar flares and Coronal Mass Ejections (CMEs), releases significant amounts of radiation that can pose risks to human health. While Earth's atmosphere and magnetic field offer substantial protection, certain populations, such as astronauts and high-altitude pilots, are more vulnerable to increased radiation exposure. This chapter delves into the types of radiation associated with solar activity, the potential health effects of increased radiation exposure, and the implications for both space exploration and aviation.

Types of Solar Radiation

Solar radiation encompasses a range of electromagnetic waves and energetic particles emitted by the sun. The key components relevant to human health include:

Electromagnetic Radiation

- Ultraviolet (UV) Radiation: UV radiation is categorized into three types based on wavelength: UVA, UVB, and UVC. While UVC is mostly absorbed by the Earth's atmosphere, UVA and UVB can reach the surface and affect skin health, contributing to conditions like sunburn and skin cancer.
- X-Rays and Gamma Rays: Solar flares emit X-rays and gamma rays, which are high-energy electromagnetic waves capable of penetrating deep into tissues and causing cellular damage.

Particulate Radiation

- Protons and Electrons: Solar energetic particles (SEPs) primarily consist of high-energy protons and electrons. These particles are accelerated by solar flares and CMEs and can penetrate biological tissues, causing ionization and molecular damage.
- Heavy Ions: Although less abundant than protons, heavy ions (such as helium nuclei) are highly energetic and can cause significant biological damage due to their high mass and charge.

Health Effects of Increased Radiation Exposure

The health effects of radiation exposure depend on the type, energy, and duration of exposure. Key health risks include:

DNA Damage and Cancer

- DNA Damage: Radiation can cause direct damage to DNA by breaking chemical bonds and creating free radicals, leading to mutations and disruptions in cellular function.
- Cancer Risk: The primary long-term health risk of radiation exposure is an increased risk of cancer. Ionizing radiation can induce genetic mutations that accumulate over time, potentially leading to malignancies. Populations exposed to higher levels of radiation, such as astronauts and pilots, have an elevated risk of developing cancer.

Acute Radiation Syndrome

- Symptoms: High doses of radiation over a short period can cause acute radiation syndrome (ARS), characterized by nausea, vomiting, fatigue, and more severe symptoms such as skin burns, hemorrhage, and organ failure at higher doses.

- Mechanism: ARS occurs due to the rapid destruction of rapidly dividing cells, particularly in the bone marrow, gastrointestinal tract, and skin.

Cardiovascular and Neurological Effects

- Cardiovascular Health: Radiation exposure can increase the risk of cardiovascular disease by damaging blood vessels and heart tissue. Studies on atomic bomb survivors and radiation therapy patients have shown increased incidences of heart disease and stroke.
- Neurological Health: High levels of radiation can affect the central nervous system, leading to cognitive impairment and increased risk of neurodegenerative diseases. This is particularly relevant for astronauts on long-duration missions, who are exposed to both galactic cosmic rays and solar radiation.

Implications for Space Exploration:

Astronauts and Space Missions

- Increased Exposure: Astronauts are exposed to higher levels of radiation in space due to the lack of atmospheric protection and the presence of galactic cosmic rays and solar energetic particles. This exposure increases significantly during solar flares and CMEs.

- Protective Measures: NASA and other space agencies employ various protective measures to mitigate radiation risks, including spacecraft shielding, mission planning to avoid solar maximum periods, and potential pharmaceutical countermeasures to protect against radiation damage.

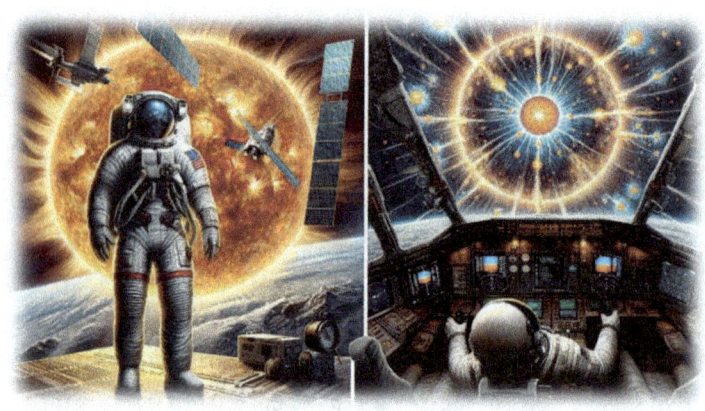

Long-Duration Missions

- Mars Missions: Future missions to Mars pose significant radiation challenges due to the long duration and limited protective shielding available en route and on the Martian surface. Strategies under consideration include improved spacecraft shielding, habitat construction using Martian regolith, and the development of advanced pharmaceuticals to mitigate radiation effects.

Implications for Aviation:

High-Altitude Pilots and Passengers

- Increased Exposure at Altitude: Pilots and passengers on high-altitude flights are exposed to higher levels of cosmic radiation compared to those at ground level. During solar storms, this exposure can increase significantly, posing potential health risks.
- Monitoring and Mitigation: Aviation authorities monitor solar activity and provide guidelines to minimize radiation exposure during flights, such as adjusting flight paths and altitudes. Airlines may also implement measures to reduce exposure, such as limiting flight durations for crew members.

Protective Measures and Future Research:

Spacecraft and Habitat Shielding

- Shielding Materials: Advances in shielding materials, such as polyethylene and other hydrogen-rich compounds, offer improved protection against radiation. Research is ongoing to develop more effective and lightweight shielding solutions for spacecraft and habitats.

- Water and Regolith Shielding: Using water and planetary regolith as shielding materials is being explored for long-duration missions. These materials can provide significant protection against both solar and cosmic radiation.

Pharmaceutical Countermeasures

- Radioprotective Agents: Researchers are investigating various compounds that can mitigate the effects of radiation exposure. These include antioxidants, anti-inflammatory agents, and compounds that enhance DNA repair mechanisms.
- Gene Therapy: Emerging research in gene therapy holds promise for protecting astronauts from radiation-induced damage by enhancing their natural protective mechanisms.

Monitoring and Early Warning Systems

- Radiation Monitoring: Continuous monitoring of radiation levels in space and at high altitudes is essential for protecting astronauts and aviation personnel. Advanced sensors and dosimeters are used to track exposure in real-time.
- Early Warning Systems: Early warning systems for solar flares and CMEs allow for timely protective measures to be implemented, such as adjusting flight paths or seeking shelter in

shielded areas of spacecraft.

This chapter has explored the various types of solar radiation associated with geomagnetic storms and their potential health effects on humans. While Earth's atmosphere provides substantial protection, certain populations, such as astronauts and high-altitude pilots, are more vulnerable to increased radiation exposure. Understanding these risks and developing effective protective measures is crucial for ensuring the safety of those exposed to higher radiation levels.

As we continue to examine the broader implications of solar activity on human health, the subsequent chapters will focus on oxidative stress, immune responses, and potential protective measures. By integrating insights from various scientific disciplines, we aim to provide a comprehensive understanding of the complex interactions between solar activity and our biological systems.

10 CASE STUDIES AND RESEARCH DATA

To understand the impact of geomagnetic storms on human health, examining case studies and research data is essential.

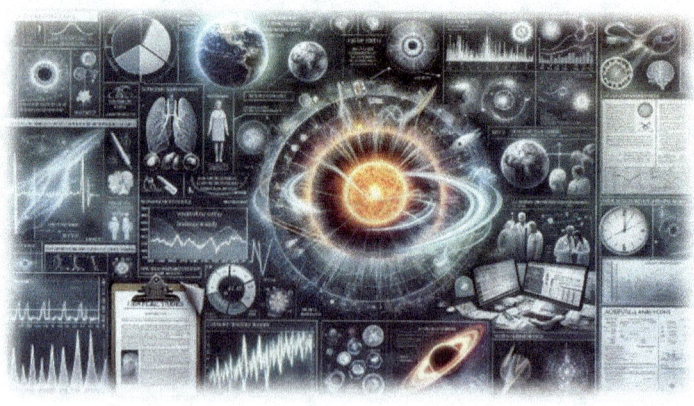

These real-world examples and scientific investigations provide insights into the potential correlations between solar activity and various health outcomes. This chapter presents a detailed review of significant case studies and epidemiological research, highlighting key findings and their implications for public health.

The Carrington Event (1859)

The Carrington Event remains the most powerful geomagnetic storm on record. Named after British astronomer Richard Carrington, who observed the associated solar flare, this event provides a historical benchmark for understanding the potential severity of geomagnetic storms.

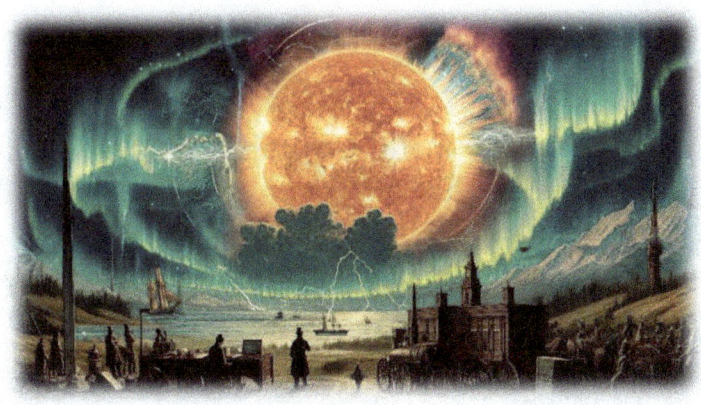

- Impact on Technology: During the Carrington Event, telegraph systems across Europe and North America failed, with some telegraph operators experiencing electric shocks. Aurora displays were visible as far south as the Caribbean, indicating the widespread impact of the geomagnetic storm.

- Health Implications: Although detailed health records from this period are scarce, the magnitude of the event suggests that any similar future occurrence could have significant health impacts, particularly given modern society's reliance on technology.

The 1989 Quebec Blackout

In March 1989, a powerful geomagnetic storm caused a nine-hour blackout in Quebec, Canada, highlighting the vulnerability of power grids to geomagnetic disturbances.

- Technological Disruptions: The storm induced geomagnetically induced currents (GICs) in power lines, leading to transformer failures and widespread power outages.
- Health Implications: Studies conducted during this period reported an increase in hospital admissions for cardiovascular issues, such as heart attacks and strokes, suggesting a possible link between geomagnetic activity and cardiovascular health.

The Halloween Storms (2003)

The Halloween Storms in late October 2003 were a series of intense geomagnetic storms caused by multiple CMEs. These storms provided valuable data on the impacts of solar activity.

- Technological Disruptions: The storms disrupted satellite communications, caused power outages in Sweden, and resulted in auroras visible as far south as Texas.
- Health Implications: Research during this period indicated an increase in psychiatric hospital admissions and cardiovascular events, further supporting the hypothesis that geomagnetic storms can influence human health.

Epidemiological Research

Epidemiological studies have explored the correlations between geomagnetic activity and various health outcomes. These studies use large datasets and statistical analysis to identify potential links between solar activity and health issues.

Cardiovascular Health

- Heart Attacks and Strokes: Numerous studies

have reported a higher incidence of heart attacks and strokes during periods of increased geomagnetic activity. For example, a study published in the *American Journal of Epidemiology* found a significant association between geomagnetic storms and increased mortality due to cardiovascular causes.

- Mechanisms: The proposed mechanisms for these effects include increased blood clotting, changes in heart rate variability, and elevated oxidative stress during geomagnetic storms.

Neurological and Psychiatric Health

- Mood Disorders: Research has shown that geomagnetic activity is associated with higher rates of mood disorders, such as depression and anxiety. A study in the *Journal of Affective Disorders* reported increased incidences of depressive episodes during periods of high geomagnetic activity.

- Psychiatric Admissions: Several studies have found a correlation between geomagnetic storms and increased psychiatric hospital admissions. For instance, research conducted in Russia and the UK observed spikes in psychiatric admissions during geomagnetic storms, suggesting a potential link between solar activity and mental health.

Sleep Disorders

- Sleep Patterns: Geomagnetic storms have been linked to disruptions in sleep patterns. Studies have reported changes in sleep quality and duration during periods of high geomagnetic activity, likely due to reduced melatonin production.
- Mechanisms: The hypothesized mechanisms include electromagnetic interference with the pineal gland and increased physiological stress during geomagnetic storms.

Key Findings and Implications

The case studies and epidemiological research reviewed in this chapter highlight several key findings and their implications for public health:

- Increased Health Risks: Geomagnetic storms are associated with increased risks of cardiovascular events, mood disorders, psychiatric admissions, and sleep disturbances.
- Vulnerable Populations: Certain populations, such as those with pre-existing cardiovascular or psychiatric conditions, may be more vulnerable to the health effects of geomagnetic storms.
- Public Health Preparedness: Understanding the potential health impacts of geomagnetic storms can inform public health preparedness and

response strategies. This includes developing guidelines for at-risk populations and improving monitoring and early warning systems for solar activity.

Mechanisms and Hypotheses

Understanding the mechanisms through which geomagnetic storms affect health is crucial for developing effective protective measures. Several hypotheses have been proposed:

-       Electromagnetic Field Interactions: Geomagnetic storms generate fluctuations in the Earth's magnetic field, which can interact with the human body's electromagnetic fields. These interactions may disrupt physiological processes, leading to health effects.
- Oxidative Stress and Inflammation: Increased geomagnetic activity can induce oxidative stress and inflammatory responses in the body, contributing to cardiovascular and neurological conditions.
- Autonomic Nervous System: Geomagnetic activity may affect the autonomic nervous system, influencing heart rate variability, blood pressure, and stress responses.

This chapter has provided a detailed review of significant case studies and epidemiological research on the health impacts of geomagnetic storms. The findings highlight the potential risks to cardiovascular, neurological, and psychiatric health, as well as the importance of public health preparedness.

As we continue to explore the broader implications of solar activity on human health, the subsequent chapters will focus on oxidative stress, immune responses, and potential protective measures. By integrating insights from various scientific disciplines, we aim to provide a comprehensive understanding of the complex interactions between solar activity and our biological systems.

11 PROTECTIVE MEASURES AND FUTURE RESEARCH

Understanding the potential health impacts of geomagnetic storms and solar activity on human physiology is crucial for developing effective protective measures. As our reliance on technology increases and space exploration advances, safeguarding human health against these environmental factors becomes even more important. This chapter explores various protective measures and highlights areas for future research to mitigate the risks associated with solar activity.

Spacecraft and Habitat Shielding

For astronauts and future space missions, effective shielding is vital to protect against increased radiation exposure during solar flares and geomagnetic storms.

- Material Advancements: Advances in shielding materials, such as polyethylene and other hydrogen-rich compounds, offer improved protection against radiation. These materials are effective at absorbing high-energy particles, reducing the risk of radiation-induced health effects.
- Water and Regolith Shielding: Utilizing water and planetary regolith (soil) as shielding materials is a promising strategy for long-duration missions. Water provides excellent radiation protection, and using local regolith for habitat construction can offer substantial shielding on planetary surfaces, such as the Moon or Mars.

Pharmaceutical Countermeasures

Developing pharmaceutical agents to mitigate the effects of radiation exposure is a crucial area of research.

- Radioprotective Agents: Compounds such as antioxidants, anti-inflammatory agents, and molecules that enhance DNA repair mechanisms can help protect against radiation damage. Research into these agents aims to reduce the risk of cancer, cardiovascular disease, and neurological damage in astronauts and high-altitude pilots.

- Gene Therapy: Emerging research in gene therapy holds potential for enhancing natural protective mechanisms against radiation. By modifying genes involved in DNA repair and oxidative stress response, it may be possible to increase resistance to radiation-induced damage.

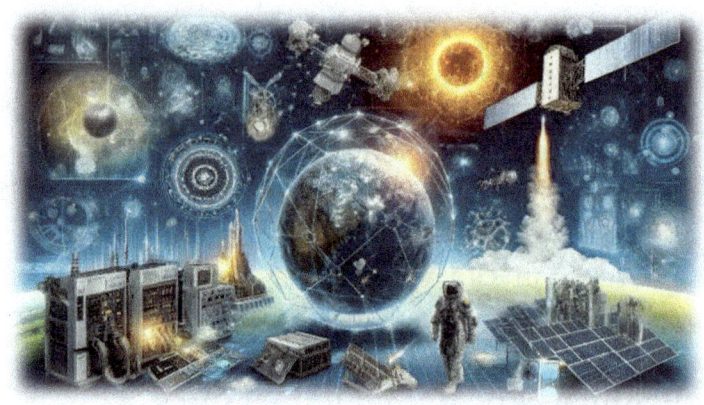

Monitoring and Early Warning Systems

Continuous monitoring of solar activity and radiation levels is essential for protecting vulnerable populations.

- Radiation Monitoring: Advanced sensors and dosimeters are used to track radiation exposure in real-time. These devices are crucial for astronauts, pilots, and high-altitude passengers,

providing data to make informed decisions about protective measures.
- Early Warning Systems: Early warning systems for solar flares and CMEs allow for timely implementation of protective actions. These systems can provide alerts for adjusting flight paths, seeking shelter in shielded areas of spacecraft, and taking other precautionary measures.

Personal Protective Measures

Individuals, particularly those in high-risk professions, can take steps to protect themselves from the effects of geomagnetic storms.

- Avoiding High-Exposure Activities: During periods of high geomagnetic activity, reducing time spent in high-altitude flights or spacewalks can minimize exposure to radiation.
- Health Monitoring: Regular health check-ups and monitoring for cardiovascular and neurological symptoms can help detect and manage potential health effects early.

Future Research Directions

While significant progress has been made in understanding and mitigating the health impacts of geomagnetic storms, several areas require

further research:
Mechanisms of Action

Understanding the precise mechanisms through which geomagnetic storms affect human health is critical for developing targeted protective measures.

- Electromagnetic Field Interactions: Research into how geomagnetic fluctuations interact with the human body's electromagnetic fields can provide insights into the physiological processes affected by solar activity.
- Oxidative Stress and Inflammation: Investigating the pathways through which geomagnetic activity induces oxidative stress and inflammatory responses can help identify potential therapeutic targets.

Long-Term Health Effects

Longitudinal studies are needed to assess the long-term health impacts of repeated exposure to geomagnetic storms and radiation.

- Epidemiological Studies: Large-scale epidemiological studies can help identify correlations between geomagnetic activity and health outcomes, providing a broader understanding of the risks.

- Astronaut Health: Monitoring the health of astronauts over extended periods can provide valuable data on the long-term effects of space radiation and geomagnetic storms, informing future mission planning and protective strategies.

Technological Innovations

Developing new technologies to protect against the effects of solar activity is an ongoing priority.

- Advanced Shielding Materials: Research into novel materials and construction techniques for spacecraft and habitats can enhance radiation protection without significantly increasing weight and cost.
- Wearable Technology: Personal wearable devices that monitor radiation exposure and provide real-time health data can empower individuals to take proactive measures to protect their health.

Public Health Preparedness

Improving public health preparedness for geomagnetic storms is essential for mitigating risks to the general population.

- Public Awareness Campaigns: Educating the public about the potential health impacts of geomagnetic storms and promoting protective behaviors can reduce vulnerability.

- Healthcare System Readiness: Ensuring that healthcare systems are equipped to handle potential increases in cardiovascular and neurological cases during geomagnetic storms can enhance resilience.

This chapter has explored various protective measures and future research directions to mitigate the health impacts of geomagnetic storms and solar activity. From advanced shielding for astronauts to pharmaceutical countermeasures and early warning systems, a multi-faceted approach is essential for safeguarding human health. Continued research into the mechanisms of action, long-term health effects, and technological innovations will further enhance our ability to protect against these environmental risks.

As we conclude this comprehensive exploration of the interactions between solar activity and human health, it is clear that understanding and mitigating these impacts is crucial for both current and future generations. By integrating insights from various scientific disciplines and continuing to advance our knowledge, we can ensure a safer and healthier future in the face of the dynamic and powerful forces of our nearest star.

12 TECHNOLOGICAL INNOVATIONS FOR RESILIENCE: FROM SATELLITES TO WEARABLES

As our understanding of the impacts of solar activity and geomagnetic storms on human health and technological infrastructure deepens, the development of innovative technologies becomes crucial for enhancing resilience. This chapter explores a range of technological advancements designed to mitigate the effects of space weather, from sophisticated satellite systems to wearable health devices. These innovations not only help protect critical infrastructure but also empower individuals to manage their exposure to geomagnetic disturbances.

Satellite Technology and Space Weather Monitoring

Satellites play a pivotal role in monitoring solar activity and predicting geomagnetic storms. Advances in satellite technology have significantly improved our ability to understand and respond to space weather events.

Advanced Satellite Instruments

1. Solar Observatories: Satellites equipped with advanced instruments, such as the Solar and Heliospheric Observatory (SOHO) and the Solar Dynamics Observatory (SDO), provide continuous monitoring of the sun. These observatories capture high-resolution images and data on solar flares, CMEs, and other solar phenomena, enabling scientists to track and predict space weather events.

2. Magnetometers and Particle Detectors: Satellites like the GOES (Geostationary Operational Environmental Satellites) series are equipped with magnetometers and particle detectors that measure the intensity of geomagnetic storms and the flux of energetic particles. These instruments provide real-time data on space weather conditions, which are essential for forecasting and mitigation efforts.

Early Warning Systems

1. Real-Time Alerts: Advanced satellite systems can issue real-time alerts for impending geomagnetic storms, giving operators of critical infrastructure time to implement protective measures. These alerts are crucial for power grid operators, satellite communication providers, and aviation authorities.

2. Data Integration and Analysis: Integration of satellite data with ground-based observations and computer models enhances the accuracy of space weather forecasts. Sophisticated algorithms analyze data from multiple sources to predict the onset, duration, and intensity of geomagnetic storms.

Protecting Critical Infrastructure

Technological innovations are vital for safeguarding critical infrastructure, such as power grids, communication networks, and navigation systems, against the impacts of geomagnetic storms.

Power Grid Protection

1. Geomagnetically Induced Current (GIC)

Mitigation: Technologies such as GIC monitoring systems and advanced transformer designs help protect power grids from geomagnetic storm-induced currents. These systems detect abnormal currents and enable operators to take preventive actions, such as adjusting load distributions and temporarily shutting down vulnerable components.

2. Resilient Grid Architecture: Developing more resilient grid architectures, including decentralized and microgrid systems, enhances the ability to isolate and manage disruptions caused by geomagnetic storms. These innovations increase the robustness of power supply and reduce the risk of widespread blackouts.

Satellite and Communication System Resilience

1. Hardened Satellite Electronics: Innovations in satellite design, including the use of radiation-hardened electronics, improve the resilience of satellites to solar radiation and energetic particles. These enhancements extend the operational lifespan of satellites and reduce the likelihood of failures during geomagnetic storms.

2. Redundant Communication Networks:

Implementing redundant communication networks ensures that critical communication systems remain operational during space weather events. This includes the use of multiple satellite constellations, ground-based communication links, and alternative frequencies to maintain connectivity.

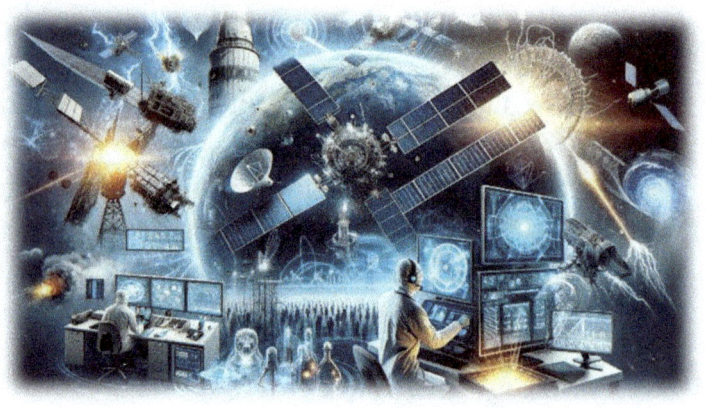

Navigation System Accuracy

1. Enhanced GPS Resilience: Technologies such as advanced signal processing algorithms and multi-frequency receivers enhance the resilience of GPS systems to geomagnetic disturbances. These innovations improve the accuracy and reliability of navigation signals during geomagnetic storms.

2.   Alternative   Navigation   Systems:

Developing alternative navigation systems, such as the European Galileo system and Russia's GLONASS, provides redundancy and reduces reliance on a single system. This enhances global navigation resilience and ensures continuous service during space weather events.

Wearable Technology for Personal Health Monitoring

Wearable health devices are emerging as valuable tools for monitoring and managing the physiological impacts of geomagnetic storms on individuals. These devices provide real-time data on various health parameters, enabling proactive health management.

Radiation Exposure Monitoring

1. Personal Dosimeters: Wearable dosimeters measure an individual's exposure to ionizing radiation. These devices are particularly useful for astronauts, high-altitude pilots, and passengers, providing real-time data on radiation levels and alerting users to take protective actions when necessary.

2. Smart Clothing: Integrating radiation sensors into clothing offers continuous monitoring of radiation exposure. Smart clothing

can be designed to provide alerts and recommendations for minimizing exposure, enhancing personal safety during geomagnetic storms.

Heart Rate Variability (HRV) Monitoring

1. Wearable HRV Sensors: Devices such as smartwatches and chest straps equipped with HRV sensors monitor heart rate variability, a key indicator of autonomic nervous system function and stress levels. These devices help individuals track their physiological responses to geomagnetic storms and manage stress effectively.

2. Health Apps: Mobile applications that sync with wearable HRV sensors offer insights into heart rate patterns, stress levels, and overall health. These apps provide personalized recommendations for maintaining optimal health during periods of high geomagnetic activity.

Sleep and Mood Tracking

1. Sleep Monitors: Wearable sleep monitors track sleep patterns, including duration and quality. These devices help individuals identify disruptions in sleep caused by geomagnetic

storms and implement strategies to improve sleep hygiene.

2. Mood Tracking Apps: Mobile apps that track mood and emotional well-being can help users recognize patterns and correlations between geomagnetic activity and their mental health. These apps offer tools for managing mood and reducing the impact of space weather on psychological well-being.

Future Innovations and Research Directions

The field of technological innovations for resilience to space weather is continually evolving. Future research and development will focus on enhancing existing technologies and exploring new solutions to mitigate the impacts of geomagnetic storms.

Advanced Shielding Materials

1. Nanotechnology: Research into nanotechnology-based shielding materials offers the potential for highly effective radiation protection with minimal weight. These materials could be used in spacecraft, satellites, and personal protective equipment.

2. Hybrid Materials: Developing hybrid

shielding materials that combine multiple protective properties, such as radiation absorption and mechanical strength, can provide enhanced protection for critical infrastructure and individuals.

Artificial Intelligence and Machine Learning

1. Predictive Modeling: Artificial intelligence (AI) and machine learning algorithms can analyze vast datasets to improve the accuracy of space weather predictions. These technologies can identify patterns and trends, enabling more precise forecasting of geomagnetic storms.

2. Automated Response Systems: AI-driven automated response systems can manage critical infrastructure during geomagnetic storms, making real-time adjustments to protect against disruptions. These systems enhance resilience by reducing human error and improving response times.

Interdisciplinary Collaboration

1. Cross-Disciplinary Research: Collaboration between space scientists, engineers, healthcare professionals, and data scientists is essential for developing comprehensive solutions to the

challenges posed by geomagnetic storms. Interdisciplinary research can integrate diverse perspectives and expertise, leading to innovative technologies and strategies.

2. Global Cooperation: International collaboration in space weather monitoring and technology development can enhance global resilience. Sharing data, resources, and best practices across countries ensures a coordinated and effective response to space weather events.

Technological innovations are at the forefront of our efforts to enhance resilience to the impacts of solar activity and geomagnetic storms. From advanced satellite systems that provide early warnings to wearable devices that monitor personal health, these technologies play a critical role in protecting both infrastructure and individuals.

As our understanding of space weather continues to grow, so too will the development of new and innovative solutions. By embracing technological advancements and fostering interdisciplinary and international collaboration, we can better navigate the challenges posed by our dynamic sun. These efforts will ensure a safer, more resilient future in the face of the powerful forces of space weather.

Aeron P. White

13 INTEGRATING SCIENCES FOR BETTER UNDERSTANDING

The study of solar activity and its impacts on human health, technology, and society is inherently interdisciplinary. Understanding the complex interactions between solar phenomena and Earth's systems requires the integration of knowledge from diverse scientific disciplines, including astrophysics, atmospheric science, biology, medicine, engineering, and social sciences. This chapter explores the benefits of an interdisciplinary approach, highlights key areas of integration, and discusses how collaboration across fields can lead to a more comprehensive understanding and effective mitigation strategies.

The Need for Interdisciplinary Collaboration

Solar activity and its effects span multiple scientific domains. Each discipline offers unique insights and methodologies that, when combined, provide a more holistic view of the phenomena and their impacts. The interdisciplinary approach is essential for several reasons:

1. Complex Interactions: Solar activity affects Earth's magnetosphere, atmosphere, and biosphere in interconnected ways. Understanding these interactions requires expertise from various fields.
2. Comprehensive Risk Assessment: Assessing the full scope of risks posed by geomagnetic storms involves examining technological, health, and societal dimensions, necessitating a collaborative approach.
3. Innovative Solutions: Cross-disciplinary collaboration fosters innovation by combining different perspectives and techniques, leading to more effective solutions for mitigating the impacts of space weather.

Key Areas of Integration

Astrophysics and Space Weather Prediction

1. Solar Observation: Astrophysicists study

the sun's behavior, including solar flares and CMEs, using ground-based telescopes and space-based observatories. Their findings are critical for predicting space weather events.

2. Data Sharing and Modeling: Collaboration between astrophysicists and atmospheric scientists enhances the accuracy of space weather models. Shared data from satellites and observatories inform models that predict the timing, intensity, and potential impacts of geomagnetic storms.

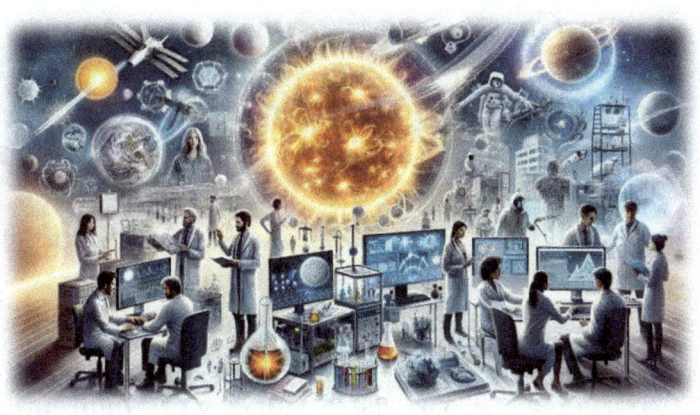

Atmospheric Science and Climate Research

1. Atmospheric Chemistry: Atmospheric scientists investigate how geomagnetic storms influence atmospheric chemistry, including the production of reactive nitrogen species and

ozone depletion. These studies help assess the broader climatic impacts of solar activity.

2. Climate Models: Integrating solar activity data into climate models allows researchers to explore potential links between solar variability and climate patterns. This interdisciplinary effort enhances our understanding of the sun's role in long-term climate change.

Biology and Medicine

1. Human Physiology: Biologists and medical researchers study the effects of geomagnetic storms on human health, including cardiovascular, neurological, and hormonal impacts. This research is vital for developing protective measures and medical interventions.

2. Radiation Effects: Collaboration between space scientists and medical researchers helps assess the health risks of increased radiation exposure during geomagnetic storms, particularly for astronauts and high-altitude pilots. This interdisciplinary work informs the design of protective technologies and health guidelines.

Engineering and Technology

1. Infrastructure Protection: Engineers design technologies to protect critical infrastructure,

such as power grids and communication networks, from the effects of geomagnetic storms. Collaborating with space scientists ensures these technologies are based on accurate space weather forecasts.

2. Innovation in Shielding: Materials scientists and engineers work together to develop advanced shielding materials for spacecraft and satellites, enhancing their resilience to solar radiation. This interdisciplinary effort combines knowledge of material properties with space weather dynamics.

Social Sciences and Public Policy

1. Risk Communication: Social scientists study how to effectively communicate the risks of geomagnetic storms to the public and policymakers. Their work ensures that information is accessible, accurate, and actionable.

2. Policy Development: Collaboration between scientists, engineers, and policy experts informs the creation of regulations and policies aimed at mitigating the impacts of space weather. This interdisciplinary approach ensures that policies are grounded in scientific evidence and technological feasibility.

Enhanced Understanding

1. Holistic Perspective: Integrating insights from various disciplines provides a more comprehensive understanding of the complex interactions between solar activity and Earth's systems. This holistic perspective is crucial for addressing multifaceted challenges.

2. Improved Predictions: Collaborative efforts improve the accuracy of space weather predictions by incorporating data and methodologies from different fields. This leads to better preparedness and response strategies.

Innovative Solutions

1. Cross-Pollination of Ideas: Interdisciplinary collaboration fosters the exchange of ideas and techniques, leading to innovative solutions. For example, combining knowledge from materials science and astrophysics can result in advanced shielding technologies for space missions.

2. Integrated Approaches: Addressing the impacts of geomagnetic storms requires integrated approaches that consider technological, health, and societal dimensions. Interdisciplinary teams can develop comprehensive strategies that address all aspects of the problem.

Effective Communication and Policy

1. Public Engagement: Interdisciplinary collaboration enhances the effectiveness of public education and outreach efforts. By incorporating insights from social sciences, communication strategies can be tailored to different audiences, improving public awareness and understanding.

2. Informed Policy-Making: Policies informed by interdisciplinary research are more likely to be effective and feasible. Collaboration between scientists, engineers, and policymakers ensures that regulations and guidelines are based on the best available evidence and technological capabilities.

The National Space Weather Strategy

1. Collaborative Framework: The National Space Weather Strategy in the United States is an example of an interdisciplinary initiative that brings together federal agencies, research institutions, and private sector stakeholders to address the challenges posed by space weather.

2. Integrated Planning: The strategy includes components focused on improving space weather forecasting, protecting critical infrastructure, and enhancing public

preparedness, demonstrating the benefits of a coordinated, interdisciplinary approach.

The European Space Agency's Space Weather Coordination Centre (SSCC)

1. Multi-Disciplinary Collaboration: The SSCC involves collaboration between astrophysicists, engineers, and communication specialists to monitor and predict space weather events. This interdisciplinary effort enhances Europe's capacity to respond to geomagnetic storms.

2. Research and Development: The SSCC supports research and development projects that integrate knowledge from various disciplines to develop innovative solutions for mitigating the impacts of space weather.

Citizen Science Projects

1. Public Participation: Citizen science projects, such as the Aurorasaurus project, involve the public in collecting data on space weather phenomena. These initiatives foster collaboration between scientists and non-experts, enhancing data collection and public engagement.

2. Educational Outreach: By involving the public in scientific research, citizen science

projects also serve an educational purpose, increasing awareness and understanding of space weather and its impacts.

Strengthening Collaboration Networks

1. Research Consortia: Establishing research consortia that bring together experts from different fields can facilitate ongoing collaboration and the sharing of resources and knowledge.

2. International Cooperation: Promoting international cooperation in space weather research can enhance global resilience. Sharing data, best practices, and technological advancements across countries can lead to more effective solutions.

Expanding Interdisciplinary Training

1. Educational Programs: Developing educational programs that emphasize interdisciplinary training can prepare the next generation of scientists, engineers, and policymakers to address the complex challenges of space weather.

2. Professional Development: Providing opportunities for professionals to gain interdisciplinary skills and knowledge through workshops, conferences, and collaborative

projects can enhance their ability to contribute to integrated research and solutions.

Fostering Innovation through Interdisciplinary Research

1. Funding and Support: Increasing funding and support for interdisciplinary research projects can drive innovation. Grant programs that encourage collaboration across disciplines can stimulate the development of new technologies and strategies.

2. Collaborative Platforms: Creating platforms for interdisciplinary collaboration, such as virtual labs and research networks, can facilitate communication and cooperation among researchers from different fields.

The interdisciplinary approach is essential for understanding and mitigating the impacts of solar activity and geomagnetic storms. By integrating knowledge and methodologies from diverse scientific disciplines, we can achieve a more comprehensive understanding of these phenomena and develop innovative solutions to address their effects on human health, technology, and society.

As we move forward, fostering collaboration, expanding interdisciplinary training, and supporting innovative research will be crucial for building resilience to space weather. By embracing the interdisciplinary approach, we can ensure a safer and more informed future, capable of navigating the challenges and opportunities presented by our dynamic and powerful sun.

14 BROADER IMPLICATIONS AND SOCIETAL IMPACT

The potential health impacts of geomagnetic storms and solar activity extend beyond individual health concerns to broader societal implications. These environmental phenomena can influence public health, economic stability, and the overall functioning of modern society. This chapter explores the wider ramifications of solar activity, highlighting the interconnectedness of technology, health, and societal resilience.

Public Health Implications

Geomagnetic storms can have significant public health implications, particularly for vulnerable populations.

Increased Healthcare Demand

- Cardiovascular and Neurological Health: As discussed in previous chapters, geomagnetic storms can exacerbate cardiovascular and neurological conditions. During periods of high geomagnetic activity, healthcare systems may see an increase in hospital admissions for heart attacks, strokes, and psychiatric conditions.
- Preparedness and Response: Public health agencies need to be prepared for potential surges in healthcare demand. This includes developing protocols for managing increased patient loads and ensuring that healthcare providers are aware of the potential impacts of geomagnetic storms on health.

Vulnerable Populations

- At-Risk Groups: Certain populations, such as the elderly, individuals with pre-existing cardiovascular or psychiatric conditions, and those in high-risk occupations (e.g., astronauts, high-altitude pilots), are more vulnerable to the effects of geomagnetic storms. Public health strategies should focus on protecting these groups through targeted interventions and preventive measures.
- Public Awareness: Increasing public awareness

about the health risks associated with geomagnetic storms can help individuals take proactive steps to protect themselves. Educational campaigns and public service announcements can play a key role in disseminating this information.

Economic Impact

Geomagnetic storms can have substantial economic repercussions, particularly due to their impact on critical infrastructure.

Power Grids and Energy Systems

- Grid Vulnerability: Power grids are highly susceptible to geomagnetically induced currents (GICs), which can cause transformer damage and widespread power outages. The economic cost of these disruptions can be significant, affecting businesses, healthcare facilities, and daily life.
- Mitigation Strategies: Investing in technologies to protect power grids, such as improved transformer design, real-time monitoring systems, and grid management protocols, can reduce the economic impact of geomagnetic storms.

Communication and Navigation Systems

- Satellite Disruptions: Geomagnetic storms can disrupt satellite communications and GPS systems, leading to economic losses in sectors that rely on these technologies, including aviation, maritime navigation, and emergency services.
- Resilience Measures: Enhancing the resilience of satellite and communication systems through improved shielding, redundancy, and backup systems can mitigate these risks.

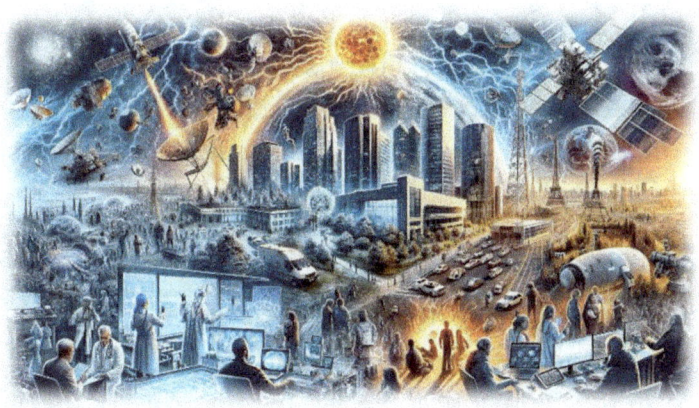

Societal Resilience

Building societal resilience to geomagnetic storms involves a comprehensive approach that includes infrastructure protection, public health preparedness, and community awareness.

Infrastructure Protection

- Critical Infrastructure: Protecting critical infrastructure, such as power grids, communication networks, and transportation systems, is essential for maintaining societal stability during geomagnetic storms. This includes implementing engineering solutions, developing contingency plans, and conducting regular infrastructure assessments.
- Research and Development: Continued investment in research and development can lead to innovative solutions for mitigating the effects of geomagnetic storms on infrastructure. Collaboration between government, industry, and academia is crucial for advancing these efforts.

Public Health Preparedness

- Healthcare Systems: Ensuring that healthcare systems are equipped to handle the potential impacts of geomagnetic storms is vital. This includes training healthcare providers, developing response protocols, and ensuring adequate resources are available.
- Emergency Preparedness: Public health agencies should integrate geomagnetic storm scenarios into emergency preparedness plans.

This includes conducting drills, establishing communication networks, and coordinating with other emergency services.

Community Awareness and Education

- Public Education Campaigns: Raising awareness about the potential impacts of geomagnetic storms and the steps individuals can take to protect themselves is crucial. Educational materials, workshops, and public service announcements can help inform the public.
- Community Engagement: Engaging communities in preparedness efforts can enhance resilience. This includes involving community leaders, schools, and local organizations in disseminating information and promoting protective measures.

Future Directions

As our understanding of the impacts of geomagnetic storms on human health and society evolves, several areas warrant further exploration:

Interdisciplinary Research

- Cross-Disciplinary Collaboration: Collaborative research involving space scientists, healthcare professionals, engineers, and social scientists can provide a holistic understanding of the impacts of geomagnetic storms and develop comprehensive mitigation strategies.

- Longitudinal Studies: Long-term studies tracking the health outcomes of individuals exposed to geomagnetic storms can provide valuable data on the chronic effects of these events.

Policy and Regulation

- Government Policies: Governments can play a crucial role in promoting resilience to geomagnetic storms through policies and regulations. This includes setting standards for infrastructure protection, funding research, and supporting public health initiatives.

- International Collaboration: Geomagnetic storms are a global phenomenon, and international collaboration is essential for addressing their impacts. Sharing data, best practices, and resources can enhance global preparedness and resilience.

Technological Innovation

- Advanced Monitoring Systems: Developing advanced monitoring and early warning systems for solar activity can help mitigate the impacts of geomagnetic storms. These systems can provide real-time data to inform protective measures.

- Protective Technologies: Investing in the development of new technologies for radiation shielding, infrastructure protection, and health monitoring can enhance resilience to geomagnetic storms.

This chapter has explored the broader implications and societal impact of geomagnetic storms, highlighting the interconnectedness of technology, health, and societal resilience. From public health preparedness to economic stability, the effects of solar activity are far-reaching and complex. Building resilience requires a comprehensive approach that includes infrastructure protection, public awareness, and continued research.

As we conclude this exploration of the interactions between solar activity and human health, it is clear that understanding and mitigating these impacts is crucial for both current and future generations. By integrating insights from various scientific disciplines and advancing our knowledge, we can ensure a safer and healthier future in the face of the dynamic and powerful forces of our nearest star.

15 SUMMARY AND FUTURE PERSPECTIVES

As we conclude our exploration of the impacts of solar activity and geomagnetic storms on human health and society, it is essential to reflect on the key findings and consider the future directions in this field. This final chapter provides a summary of the main topics discussed in the book and offers perspectives on future research, technological advancements, and policy implications.

Solar Activity and Geomagnetic Storms

- Mechanisms: Solar flares and Coronal Mass Ejections (CMEs) are primary drivers of geomagnetic storms. These solar events release vast amounts of energy and charged particles, which interact with Earth's magnetosphere, causing geomagnetic disturbances.

- Classification and Effects: Geomagnetic storms are classified based on their intensity using indices such as the Kp index. These storms can disrupt technological systems, including power grids, satellite communications, and navigation systems.

Health Impacts

- Cardiovascular Effects: Geomagnetic storms can influence heart rate variability, blood pressure, and the incidence of cardiovascular events such as heart attacks and strokes. The mechanisms include increased blood clotting and autonomic nervous system disruption.
- Neurological Effects: The nervous system is sensitive to geomagnetic activity, with potential impacts on brain wave patterns, cognitive function, mood, and mental health. Increased geomagnetic activity has been linked to higher rates of depression, anxiety, and psychiatric hospital admissions.
- Hormonal Regulation: Geomagnetic storms can disrupt the production of melatonin and serotonin, leading to sleep disturbances and mood disorders. These effects are mediated by electromagnetic field interactions and oxidative stress.
- Radiation Exposure: Increased solar radiation during geomagnetic storms poses risks,

particularly for astronauts and high-altitude pilots. Radiation exposure can lead to DNA damage, cancer, acute radiation syndrome, and cardiovascular and neurological effects.

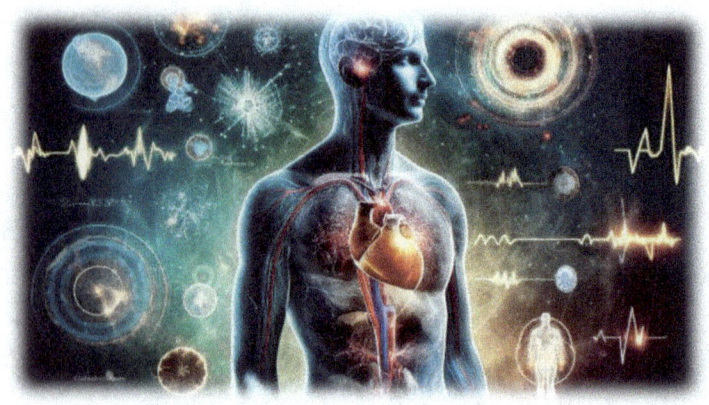

Societal and Economic Impacts

- Public Health: Geomagnetic storms can lead to increased healthcare demand, particularly for cardiovascular and neurological conditions. Public health preparedness is crucial to manage potential surges in healthcare needs.
- Economic Stability: Disruptions to power grids, communication networks, and navigation systems can have significant economic repercussions. Protecting critical infrastructure and developing resilient systems is essential for economic stability.
- Societal Resilience: Building societal resilience

involves infrastructure protection, public health preparedness, community awareness, and education. Collaborative efforts between government, industry, and academia are vital for enhancing resilience.

Research Directions

- Mechanisms of Action: Further research is needed to understand the precise mechanisms through which geomagnetic storms affect human health. This includes studying electromagnetic field interactions, oxidative stress, and inflammatory responses.
- Long-Term Health Effects: Longitudinal studies tracking the health outcomes of individuals exposed to geomagnetic storms can provide valuable data on chronic effects and inform protective strategies.
- Interdisciplinary Collaboration: Cross-disciplinary research involving space scientists, healthcare professionals, engineers, and social scientists can provide a comprehensive understanding of the impacts and develop holistic mitigation strategies.

Technological Advancements

- Advanced Shielding: Developing advanced shielding materials for spacecraft and habitats is crucial for protecting astronauts from radiation. Research into novel materials and construction techniques can enhance protection without significantly increasing weight and cost.

- Monitoring and Early Warning Systems: Enhancing monitoring and early warning systems for solar activity can mitigate the impacts of geomagnetic storms. Real-time data and alerts allow for timely protective measures.

- Wearable Technology: Personal wearable devices that monitor radiation exposure and provide real-time health data can empower individuals to take proactive steps to protect their health.

Policy Implications

- Government Policies: Governments play a crucial role in promoting resilience to geomagnetic storms through policies and regulations. This includes setting standards for infrastructure protection, funding research, and supporting public health initiatives.

- International Collaboration: Geomagnetic storms are a global phenomenon, and international collaboration is essential for addressing their impacts. Sharing data, best practices, and resources can enhance global preparedness and resilience.

- Public Awareness Campaigns: Educating the

public about the potential impacts of geomagnetic storms and promoting protective behaviors is crucial. Public education campaigns and community engagement can increase awareness and resilience.

Space Exploration and Human Health

- Mars and Beyond: Future missions to Mars and other deep-space destinations pose significant radiation challenges. Developing effective protective measures and understanding the health impacts of long-duration space travel are critical for the success of these missions.
- Health Monitoring: Continuous health monitoring of astronauts and high-altitude pilots can provide valuable data on the effects of radiation and geomagnetic storms. This data can inform protective strategies and improve health outcomes.

The exploration of the impacts of solar activity and geomagnetic storms on human health and society has highlighted the complex and far-reaching effects of these environmental phenomena. From cardiovascular and neurological health to economic stability and societal resilience, understanding and mitigating these impacts is crucial for both current and future generations.

By integrating insights from various scientific disciplines, advancing technological innovations, and promoting collaborative efforts, we can enhance our ability to protect human health and ensure a resilient society in the face of dynamic and powerful solar forces. As we look to the future, continued research, technological advancements, and informed policies will be essential for navigating the challenges and opportunities presented by our ever-changing sun.

16 EMBRACING A RESILIENT FUTURE

The journey through the impacts of solar activity and geomagnetic storms on human health and society has illuminated the profound and multifaceted ways in which our closest star influences life on Earth. As we synthesize the knowledge presented in this book, it becomes clear that preparing for and mitigating these impacts requires a multidisciplinary approach that encompasses scientific research, technological innovation, policy development, and public education.

Integrating Knowledge for Comprehensive Understanding

Understanding the impacts of solar activity involves integrating knowledge across various fields:

- Space Science and Astrophysics: Studying the mechanisms of solar flares, Coronal Mass Ejections (CMEs), and their interactions with Earth's magnetosphere provides the foundational understanding necessary to predict and monitor geomagnetic storms.
- Medical and Health Sciences: Researching the physiological and biochemical effects of geomagnetic activity on human health, particularly concerning cardiovascular, neurological, and hormonal systems, highlights the need for targeted medical interventions and preventive measures.
- Engineering and Technology: Developing advanced shielding materials, monitoring systems, and resilient infrastructure is crucial for protecting technology-dependent societies from the disruptive effects of geomagnetic storms.
- Public Health and Policy: Crafting informed policies and preparedness plans ensures that healthcare systems and public services can effectively respond to the health impacts of geomagnetic storms, safeguarding vulnerable populations and maintaining societal stability.

Embracing Technological Advancements

Technological advancements play a pivotal role

in mitigating the risks associated with solar activity:

- Shielding Innovations: Continued research into effective shielding materials for spacecraft and habitats will protect astronauts from harmful radiation, enabling safer space exploration.
- Real-Time Monitoring Systems: Enhanced monitoring and early warning systems for solar activity provide critical data that inform protective actions for both space missions and terrestrial infrastructures.
- Wearable Health Technology: Personal wearable devices that track radiation exposure and provide real-time health data empower individuals to take proactive measures to protect their health, particularly those in high-risk professions.

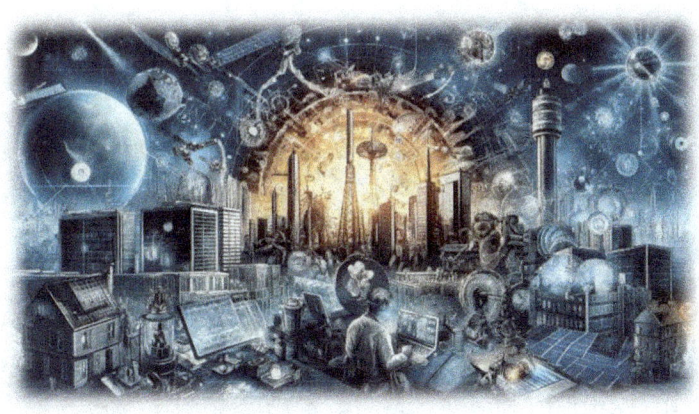

Policy and International Collaboration

Policy development and international collaboration are essential for addressing the global nature of geomagnetic storms:

- Government Initiatives: Governments must prioritize funding for research, infrastructure protection, and public health initiatives related to solar activity and geomagnetic storms. Setting regulatory standards ensures consistent and effective protection measures.
- Global Cooperation: Sharing data, resources, and best practices across nations enhances global resilience. Collaborative efforts in research and policy-making can lead to innovative solutions and a unified response to the challenges posed by solar activity.

Public Awareness and Education

Raising public awareness and fostering education about the impacts of geomagnetic storms is crucial for building a resilient society:

- Educational Campaigns: Public education campaigns can disseminate information about the potential health and technological impacts of geomagnetic storms, promoting protective

behaviors and preparedness.
- Community Engagement: Involving community leaders, schools, and local organizations in preparedness efforts can enhance resilience at the grassroots level, ensuring that individuals and communities are well-informed and equipped to respond to geomagnetic events.

Looking Ahead: A Resilient Future

As we move forward, several key areas will shape our ability to navigate the challenges and opportunities presented by solar activity:

- Continued Research: Ongoing research into the health effects of geomagnetic storms, mechanisms of action, and long-term impacts will provide the knowledge needed to develop effective interventions and protective measures.
- Technological Innovation: Advancing technologies for radiation protection, monitoring, and infrastructure resilience will play a critical role in mitigating the risks associated with solar activity.
- Policy Development: Informed policies that prioritize research funding, infrastructure protection, and public health preparedness will ensure a coordinated and effective response to geomagnetic storms.

- Global Collaboration: Strengthening international cooperation in research, policy-making, and emergency response will enhance global resilience and ensure that we are collectively prepared for the impacts of solar activity.

The influence of solar activity and geomagnetic storms on human health and society is a complex and multifaceted challenge that requires a comprehensive and collaborative approach. By integrating scientific research, technological innovation, policy development, and public education, we can build a resilient future that protects human health, safeguards technological infrastructure, and ensures societal stability in the face of the dynamic forces of our nearest star.

As we embrace this holistic approach, we are better equipped to navigate the challenges and seize the opportunities presented by our ever-changing sun. The knowledge and strategies outlined in this book provide a foundation for continued exploration, innovation, and resilience, paving the way for a safer and healthier future for all.

17 TEACHING THE PUBLIC ABOUT SOLAR ACTIVITY

Public education is a critical component in building resilience to the impacts of solar activity and geomagnetic storms. By increasing awareness and understanding of these natural phenomena, individuals and communities can better prepare for and mitigate their effects. This chapter explores the importance of educational outreach, effective strategies for teaching the public about solar activity, and examples of successful educational programs and initiatives.

The Importance of Educational Outreach

Educating the public about solar activity and its potential impacts on health, technology, and daily life is essential for several reasons:

1. Risk Awareness: Understanding the risks associated with solar activity enables individuals and communities to take proactive measures to protect themselves and their property.

2. Informed Decision-Making: Knowledge about space weather empowers people to make informed decisions, such as preparing for power outages or avoiding high-altitude flights during geomagnetic storms.

3. Enhanced Preparedness: Public education initiatives can improve community preparedness, ensuring that people know how to respond to space weather events and reduce their vulnerability.

4. Scientific Literacy: Promoting scientific literacy and curiosity about space weather can inspire future generations to pursue careers in science, technology, engineering, and mathematics (STEM).

Strategies for Effective Educational Outreach

Effective educational outreach requires a multifaceted approach that leverages various media and platforms to reach diverse audiences. Key strategies include:

School Programs and Curricula

1. Integrating Space Weather into Science Curricula: Developing and incorporating educational materials about solar activity and space weather into school science curricula can engage students and provide a foundation for understanding these phenomena. Interactive lessons, hands-on experiments, and multimedia resources can enhance learning experiences.

2. Teacher Training: Providing teachers with the knowledge and resources they need to effectively teach about solar activity is crucial. Professional development workshops and training programs can equip educators with the skills to integrate space weather topics into their classrooms.

Public Lectures and Workshops

1. Expert Talks: Hosting public lectures and talks by experts in the field of space weather can provide valuable insights and stimulate interest in the topic. These events can be held at community centers, libraries, universities, and other accessible venues.

2. Interactive Workshops: Organizing interactive workshops that involve hands-on activities and demonstrations can make learning about solar

activity more engaging. Workshops can cover topics such as building simple models of the sun, simulating geomagnetic storms, and understanding the effects of space weather on technology.

Multimedia Resources

1. Educational Videos and Documentaries: Creating and distributing educational videos and documentaries about solar activity can reach a wide audience. These resources can be shared through platforms such as YouTube, educational websites, and public television.

2. Interactive Websites and Apps: Developing interactive websites and mobile apps that provide real-time data on solar activity, educational games, and simulations can engage users and enhance their understanding of space weather.

Community Engagement and Outreach

1. Public Exhibits and Science Fairs: Participating in or organizing public exhibits and science fairs focused on space weather can raise awareness and interest. These events provide opportunities for hands-on learning and direct interaction with experts.

2. Collaborations with Local Organizations: Partnering with local organizations, such as museums, planetariums, and environmental groups, can extend the reach of educational programs. Collaborative efforts can include joint events, shared resources, and co-developed educational materials.

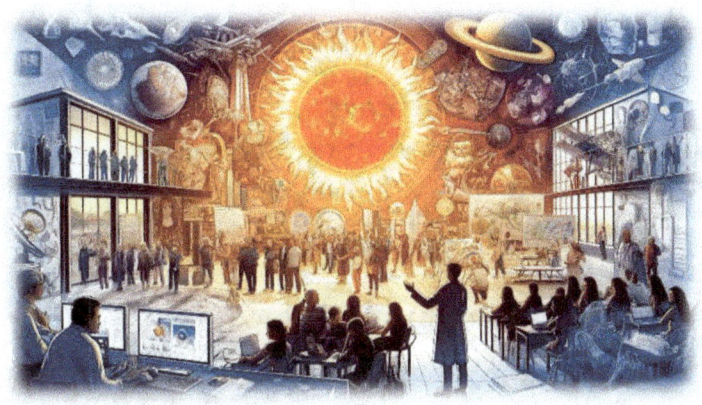

Media and Communication

1. Press Releases and Media Campaigns: Issuing press releases and conducting media campaigns during significant solar events can inform the public about potential impacts and safety measures. Collaborating with news outlets to provide accurate and timely information is essential.

2. Social Media: Leveraging social media platforms to share information about solar activity, upcoming events, and educational resources can reach a broad audience. Engaging content, such as infographics, short videos, and interactive posts, can attract and retain public interest.

Examples of Successful Educational Programs

Several educational programs and initiatives have successfully raised awareness about solar activity and its impacts. These examples highlight effective strategies and approaches:

NASA's Heliophysics Education

1. NASA's Heliophysics Division: NASA's Heliophysics Division offers a wealth of educational resources on solar activity and space weather. These include interactive websites, classroom activities, and educational videos that explain the science of the sun and its effects on Earth.

2. Space Weather Action Center (SWAC): SWAC is an interactive educational program developed by NASA that engages students in monitoring and analyzing space weather. Students use real-

time data to track solar storms and learn about their impacts on Earth.

NOAA's Space Weather Prediction Center (SWPC)

1. Educational Outreach Programs: NOAA's SWPC conducts educational outreach programs that provide information on space weather and its effects. These programs include public lectures, workshops, and resources for educators.

2. Space Weather Education Website: SWPC's website offers a variety of educational materials, including tutorials, fact sheets, and lesson plans, aimed at teaching the public and students about space weather.

European Space Agency (ESA) Education

1. ESA Education Office: The ESA Education Office provides educational resources and activities related to space weather and heliophysics. These resources are designed for students and educators across Europe.

2. Solar Weather and Space Weather Campaigns: ESA organizes educational campaigns that focus on space weather, providing interactive activities,

webinars, and resources to schools and the general public.

Future Directions for Educational Outreach

Expanding and enhancing educational outreach efforts will be crucial for increasing public understanding of solar activity and space weather. Future directions include:

Expanding Digital and Online Resources

1. Virtual Reality (VR) and Augmented Reality (AR): Developing VR and AR experiences that allow users to explore the sun and space weather phenomena in an immersive environment can enhance learning and engagement.

2. Massive Open Online Courses (MOOCs): Offering MOOCs on space weather and its impacts can reach a global audience and provide in-depth learning opportunities for interested individuals.

Inclusive and Accessible Education

1. Multilingual Resources: Creating educational materials in multiple languages can ensure that diverse communities have access to information about solar activity and space weather.

2. Inclusive Education Programs: Developing programs that cater to different learning styles and abilities can make space weather education accessible to all. This includes using visual aids, simplified explanations, and interactive tools.

Strengthening Community Partnerships

1. Community-Based Programs: Collaborating with local communities to develop tailored educational programs that address specific needs and interests can enhance relevance and impact.

2. Citizen Science Initiatives: Encouraging public participation in citizen science projects related to space weather can foster engagement and contribute valuable data to scientific research.

Educational outreach is a vital component of building resilience to the impacts of solar activity and geomagnetic storms. By raising awareness and understanding of these natural phenomena, we can empower individuals and communities to take proactive measures to protect themselves and their technology.

Effective educational outreach requires a multifaceted approach that leverages school programs, public lectures, multimedia resources, community engagement, and media communication. By exploring successful examples and adopting innovative strategies, we can enhance public understanding of space weather and promote a culture of preparedness.

As we look to the future, expanding digital and online resources, promoting inclusive and accessible education, and strengthening community partnerships will be essential for advancing educational outreach efforts. Through these collective efforts, we can ensure a more informed and resilient society, capable of navigating the challenges and opportunities presented by our dynamic and powerful sun.

18 BIBLIOGRAPHY

1. Space Science and Solar Activity
   - National Aeronautics and Space Administration (NASA). "Solar and Heliospheric Observatory (SOHO)." [Website](https://sohowww.nascom.nasa.gov/)
   - National Oceanic and Atmospheric Administration (NOAA). "Space Weather Prediction Center." [Website](https://www.swpc.noaa.gov/)
   - Lockwood, M. (2002). "The Connection Between Geomagnetic and Solar Variability." *Living Reviews in Solar Physics*, 3(2). doi:10.12942/lrsp-2002-2

2. Cardiovascular and Neurological Health
   - Stoupel, E., et al. (2002). "Cardiovascular Mortality – The Missing Link with Solar

Activity." *Journal of Basic and Clinical Physiology and Pharmacology*, 13(1), 23-38.

- Baevsky, R.M., and Berseneva, A.P. (1997). "Adaptation of Biological Systems to Geophysical Factors." Moscow: Russian Academy of Sciences.

- Otsuka, K., et al. (2001). "Geomagnetic Disturbance Associated with Decrease in Heart Rate Variability in a Subarctic Area." *Bioelectromagnetics*, 22(6), 489-495.

3. Hormonal Regulation

- Weydahl, A., et al. (2001). "Geomagnetic Activity Influences on Human Heart Rate Variability and Other Parameters of Functional State." *Bioelectromagnetics*, 22(6), 403-410.

- Chibisov, S.M., et al. (2008). "Melatonin Production in Humans During a 59-Hour Period of Geomagnetic Storms." *Biological Rhythm Research*, 39(6), 493-503.

- Burch, J.B., et al. (1999). "Geophysical Variables and Behavior: LXXVIII. Geomagnetic Indices and Human Melatonin Production." *International Journal of Biometeorology*, 43(1), 1-7.

4. Radiation Exposure

- Cucinotta, F.A., et al. (2013). "Space Radiation and Astronaut Health." *Life Sciences in Space Research*, 1, 5-18.

- Durante, M., and Cucinotta, F.A. (2011). "Physical Basis of Radiation Protection in Space Travel." *Reviews of Modern Physics*, 83(4), 1245-1281.

- National Council on Radiation Protection and Measurements (NCRP). (2006). "Information Needed to Make Radiation Protection Recommendations for Space Missions Beyond Low-Earth Orbit." NCRP Report No. 153.

5. Societal and Economic Impacts
- Boteler, D.H. (2001). "Assessment of Geomagnetic Hazard to Power Systems in Canada." *Natural Hazards*, 23, 101-120.

- Pulkkinen, A., et al. (2012). "Geomagnetic Storms: Societal Impacts and Emergency Management." *Space Weather*, 10, S04003. doi:10.1029/2011SW000765

- Oughton, E.J., et al. (2017). "A Risk Assessment Framework for the Socio-economic Impacts of Electricity Transmission Infrastructure Failure Due to Space Weather." *Risk Analysis*, 37(10), 206-221.

6. Public Health Preparedness
- Baker, D.N., et al. (2008). "Severe Space Weather Events—Understanding Societal and Economic Impacts." *National Research Council*. Washington, D.C.: National

Academies Press.

- Royal Academy of Engineering. (2013). "Extreme Space Weather: Impacts on Engineered Systems and Infrastructure." [Report](https://www.raeng.org.uk/publications/reports/space-weather-full-report)

- Centers for Disease Control and Prevention (CDC). "Public Health Preparedness Capabilities: National Standards for State and Local Planning." [Website](https://www.cdc.gov/cpr/readiness/capabilities.htm)

7. Technological Innovations and Protective Measures

- Schwadron, N.A., et al. (2010). "Space Radiation Shielding Strategies for Interplanetary Missions." *Acta Astronautica*, 67(9-10), 1190-1200.

- Townsend, L.W. (2005). "Overview of Active Methods for Shielding Spacecraft from Energetic Space Radiation." *Space Science Reviews*, 110, 145-156.

- Hellweg, C.E., and Baumstark-Khan, C. (2007). "Getting Ready for the Manned Mission to Mars: The Astronauts' Risk from Space Radiation." *Naturwissenschaften*, 94, 517-526.

8. Public Awareness and Education

- Lanzerotti, L.J. (2007). "Space Weather Effects on Communications." *Space Weather*, 5, S07002. doi:10.1029/2006SW000257

- Hapgood, M. (2012). "Preparing for the Next Space Weather Storm." *Astronomy & Geophysics*, 53(2), 2.22-2.26.

- NOAA National Centers for Environmental Information. "Space Weather Data and Products." [Website](https://www.ngdc.noaa.gov/stp/spaceweather.html)

This bibliography provides a comprehensive list of sources that cover the various aspects of solar activity and its impacts on human health and society and support the detailed information presented in this book.

The Sun's Touch

Aeron P. White